"This book is a one-of-a-kind resource for the eighty-five million American adults facing hair loss. Its up-to-the-minute summaries of science and research make it an authoritative reference tool for doctors. Yet its easy style and many personal stories give comfort and hope to patients attempting to navigate their way through the many possibilities for treatment. You only need one hair loss book—and this is it."

—Charles Salinger, M.D.

The Complete Book of

Hair Loss Answers

Your Comprehensive Guide to the Latest and Best Techniques

PETER PANAGOTACOS, M.D.
www.HairDoc.com

Elite Books

Santa Rosa, CA 95403

www.Elitebooks.biz

Library of Congress Cataloging-in-Publication Data:

Panagotacos, Peter
    The complete book of hair loss answers : your comprehensive
guide to the latest and best techniques /
Peter Panagotacos. -- 2nd ed.

    p. cm.
    ISBN 0-9720028

    1. Cosmetic Surgery. 2. Hair Loss
        2005678912

Cover and Interior design by Authors Publishing Cooperative

Illustrations by Nan Sea Love

Typeset in Colonna and Hoefler Text

Printed in USA

Second Edition

10 9 8 7 6 5 4 3 2

CONTENTS

FOREWORD

As a family practice physician, I see patients of all ages with concerns about their hair loss. There are young men with the first signs of a receding hairline, post-menopausal women with thinning hair, children with various hair loss conditions, and patients of all ages with hair loss caused by medications or other causes.

Two things have struck me about these patients. First is the deep concern they have about losing their hair. Some patients seem more concerned about losing their hair than they do about their other more serious medical conditions. Secondly, I have observed that there is a great deal of misinformation about hair loss and what can be done about it.

I have found this book to be personally informative, as well as a welcome addition to the information I can provide to my patients who are suffering from any type of hair loss condition. The book is written for the general public, but is medically accurate and at times very entertaining. My patients do not need to read the entire book, but rather can look up the information that they feel applies to their own condition, and just read a chapter or two. But many read the whole book, and thank me for loaning it to them!

I think *The Complete Book of Hair Loss Answers* is the best book out there for people who want to learn about hair loss, and what can be done about it.

Elliot Felman, M.D.
Santa Monica, California

INTRODUCTION

Did you know that the oldest dermatological prescription is an Egyptian hair loss remedy that is 5,500 years old? People have searched for answers to their hair loss concerns ever since that time.

In the early years of my dermatology medical practice, I prepared written information on hair loss for my patients, including copies of articles and books by various authors. More than ten years ago, I became one of the first to provide accurate information about hair loss on the Internet with my web site, www.hairdoc.com. Although the Internet is a wonderful resource for patient education, it has some disadvantages. I have visited dozens of hair loss web sites that feature inaccurate or incomplete information and sell dubious treatment products.

Based on my contact with my own patients, communications with other physicians, and the hundreds of emails I receive from all over the world from people who are losing their hair, it is clear to me that there is an extraordinary amount of confusion about hair loss. The general public needs a source for answers to hair loss questions, and expert advice as to which solutions really work.

This book was written to address that need.

I especially want to thank Dr. Jerry Litt for his generous help in proofreading this manuscript, and many thanks for his *Drug Eruption Reference Manual,* which I refer to regularly in my office when confronted with a patient with hair loss due to medications. I would also like to thank Dr. Alice Do, who was one of my brightest medical students, for her illustrations. I thank Gary Grossman for editing the first edition of this book, and most of all I thank all of my patients over the years, whose appreciation for my work has made my medical practice both rewarding and enjoyable.

Peter J. Panagotacos, M.D.
San Francisco, California

Preface to the Second Edition

Historically, hair transplants have been the single most common form of elective cosmetic surgery. Only with the advent of liposuction did reconstructive surgery for hair loss fall to the number two most popular spot. The need for accurate, unbiased information about available options for those concerned about receding hairlines, male and female pattern baldness (referred to medically as androgenetic alopecia) and thinning hair, will be addressed in this new, updated edition.

Since the last edition of this book, a number of promising advances have been made in follicular unit grafting, cloning, stem cell transplant, and gene therapy. More is also known about the medical treatment of hair loss. Several of the chapters in the book have been expanded or changed to reflect the latest developments in this rapidly expanding field. New drugs are added to the list of drugs that cause hair loss along with a new feature that lists the brand name.

This book is meant primarily for the individual who is concerned about losing hair now and in the future, wants to learn about the various causes, and explore the options for treatment. The informed consumer can make wise decisions and take proactive steps to handle what is a very common, but very private concern. Response to the first edition from physicians and patients alike cited the book a valuable resource for those who want help understanding their condition.

I sincerely hope this book satisfies the need many of you have for a source of up to date information on hair loss that is as unbiased as possible.

1

Why Treat Hair Loss?

A t a point in our lives while growing up, we each form a mental image of ourselves.

We develop a picture of our face and body, an image of how we think others see us. When we look in a mirror, we identify with what we see and inwardly say, "That's me." Even without a mirror, we have an idea of the image of ourselves that we project to the world.

But as a man or woman begins to lose hair, the image in the mirror no longer matches the internal self-image developed over many years. This can be disturbing, since we pretty much feel the same as before. Hair loss does not affect our physical health, but it does make us look older. When we see our reflection in the mirror, a different image confronts us. We protest, "That isn't me."

Our hair is one of the most defining aspects of our appearance. A healthy head of hair makes us look attractive, youthful, and desirable. Our appearance directly affects our own self-image, and most of us want to maintain a self-image that is youthful and healthy looking.

Our appearance also affects how we interact with other people, both in how others respond to how we look, and how our appearance affects our own self-confidence. Having a full head of hair can improve the quality of our life, our success in business relationships, and our success in romance.

But despite the fact that losing hair, and even going bald, is part of the normal process of aging, we often don't accept it. At age forty, most people feel pretty much the same as they did at age thirty, or even age twenty. Confronted with hair loss, people may begin to feel foreign to themselves and somewhat disoriented. This discomfort results in a desire to return to the former, more youthful appearance. Today there are many cosmetic, medical, and surgical options for people who really want to do something about hair loss.

Take one of my patients; I'll call him "Larry." I first met Larry in 1980, when he was thirty-five-years-old. He already had considerable frontal hair loss, but the hair on his crown and back of his head was quite dense. He was a physical fitness buff, and could not come to terms with his receding hairline. He worked out, felt pretty good, and looked great, except for his hair loss.

After considering all the options, Larry decided to have hair transplant surgery. At that time, surgical procedures for hair loss resulted in an "under construction" look for a period of time following surgery. Larry was a foreman of a crew of men who installed acoustical ceilings. It was possible for him to wear a hard hat or a baseball cap to cover his new grafts until they healed. Initially, keeping his hair transplants secret was a big concern to him. Then, after about three weeks, he began to tell his friends and co-workers about his surgery for hair loss.

There was a positive response from everyone, except for one co-worker. Larry explained to me that his co-worker, who we'll call "John," began harassing him about his hair transplants during his first month following surgery. The second month, John wanted to know if the surgery was painful, and then he wanted to know how much it cost. Soon after, I met with John, and he scheduled his own hair transplantation procedure.

People want to look the way they feel. A man or woman at age forty doesn't really expect to look twenty again, but increasingly more and more people want to keep a youthful appearance. Hair helps frame the face, and it directs attention very powerfully. Everyone has seen men with a few wispy strands of hair combed over the top of their heads in an attempt to frame their face with hair. Of course their "comb-over" just directs more attention to their hair loss, which is not the desired effect.

Although our society tends to be youth-oriented, most people with hair loss are not preoccupied with achieving a perpetually youthful appearance. In fact, many people accept their hair loss as just a fact of life. Humans have an enormous ability to adjust to imperfect situations and go on with their lives. But if you're reading this book, you probably have an interest in doing something about your hair loss.

Wanting to do something about hair loss is not just a matter of vanity. The desire to look better and have a more pleasing appearance is also a normal human attitude. Undeniably, hair loss adds years to a person's appearance. Hair loss represents to men what wrinkles do to women. And hair loss for women is even worse than wrinkles! And

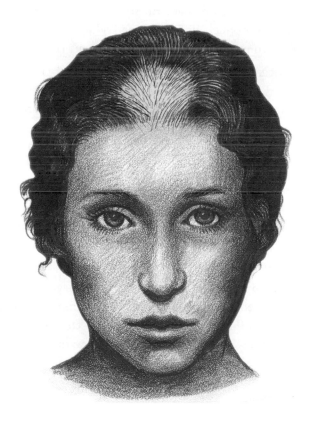

Female hair loss

while men with hair loss often state that they don't care about losing their hair, if there were some form of magic that could instantly and permanently give them a full head of hair just by wishing it, the vast majority would do just that.

In 1995, Sean Connery stated in an interview, "I don't understand men who want hair transplants." That same month, he was photographed going to a social event wearing a hairpiece. Five years later, he seemed to have accepted his baldness in his personal life. He does, however, continue to wear a hairpiece for movie roles that call for a man with a full head of hair.

The media, especially television and movies, continue to place enormous emphasis on models, actors, and actresses with hair. Women portrayed in the media, and in advertisements for almost any product, generally have full heads of hair. Entire industries are dedicated to women's hair care products and hair care styling services, all with the goal of helping women make the most of the hair they have.

The significance of hair to women in our society is so great, that women suffering chemotherapy for cancer treatment are often more emotionally devastated by their chemotherapy-induced hair loss than from their cancer.

Men's magazines rarely display a man with thinning hair, and almost never one who is bald. When the media displays an image of a desirable macho man, he is shown with a full head of hair. Unless, that is, the man is a "bad guy." Despite the increasing appearance of Hollywood talent and national sports celebrities with natural baldness or shaved heads, it still seems that when a bald man is portrayed in the media, more often than not, he is a villain.

When women were asked in a variety of surveys whether they thought men looked better bald or with hair, a majority replied that baldness did not influence their attraction to the opposite sex. Yet when shown digitally altered photos of the same men with and without hair, those same women said repeatedly that the men with hair looked more attractive to them.

2

Normal Hair Growth

Before addressing the causes and solutions to hair loss, it will be helpful to understand how hair normally grows. This is because many hair loss remedies point to aspects of normal hair growth, in particular to the shedding of hairs, as evidence of a "problem" that they can "cure." And the many causes of hair loss and various treatments become less mysterious after gaining a basic understanding of the normal cycle of hair growth.

Each strand of hair is a complex weaving of lifeless protein produced by a teardrop-shaped hair follicle. The hair follicles are made of living cells that receive nourishment entirely from the blood supply under the skin. The hair itself is made up of completely dead cells. Dead hair shaft cells cannot be "revived" to bring your dull hair back to life as claimed by many hair products.

There are hundreds of thousands of hair follicles in the skin covering almost every part of the body. Some hair follicles produce fine almost colorless "peach fuzz" hairs, and others produce thicker pigmented hair shafts. Each hair follicle is a miniature organ that grows a single hair during a phase of growth. That single hair can last for several months or several years, depending on how the follicle has been genetically programmed. Scalp hair follicles tend to have a longer growth phase than eyelash hair follicles, for example.

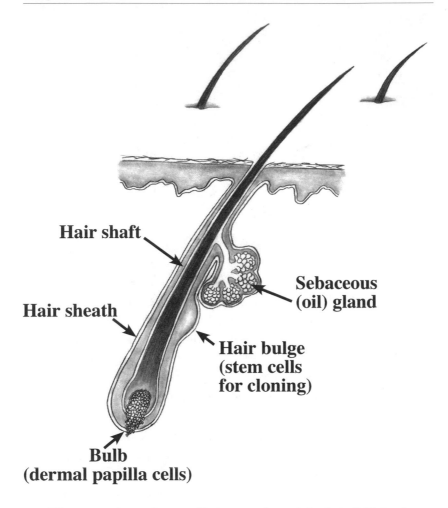

Hair shaft

Sebaceous (oil) gland

Hair sheath

Hair bulge (stem cells for cloning)

Bulb (dermal papilla cells)

There are three phases of hair growth, and the hair follicle changes significantly from phase to phase. The three phases are the anagen phase, the catagen phase, and the telogen phase.

Anagen Phase: The anagen phase is the "growing" phase of a hair follicle. It begins with a miniaturized hair follicle that may or may not have recently shed the hair it was growing during the previous growth cycle. At the beginning of the anagen phase, the hair follicle starts to grow back to full size and extend deeper into the skin. A new hair bulb is formed at the base of the follicle, and inside the hair bulb specialized dermal papilla cells begin to grow a new hair shaft. If the old hair has not been shed already, the new growing hair helps "push" the old hair out of the follicle. As the new hair grows out from the base of the follicle, it extends beyond the surface of the skin and appears as straight or curly, and with a color that can be blonde or brown or red or gray. Scalp hairs grow about one-half inch per month during the anagen phase, for a period of time typically ranging from four to six years. This is a rapid rate of cellular growth compared to most other tissues in the body.

Catagen Phase: Following the anagen phase, the hair stops growing and the hair follicle starts shrinking. This "regression" period is called the catagen phase. During the catagen phase the lower part of the hair follicle slowly disintegrates, and the hair follicle requires less nourishment from the blood supply. The structure of the hair bulb at the base of the follicle disappears, and the dermal papilla cells separate from the base of the follicle. The miniaturized hair follicle has a looser "grip" on

Hair Shedding is a normal part of the cycle of hair growth.

the hair shaft, and normal body movement, grooming, or bathing may result in the hair shaft being shed at this time. The catagen phase for scalp hair follicles lasts about two to three weeks.

Telogen Phase: After the hair follicle has stopped shrinking, it enters the telogen or "resting" phase, which lasts for another three months, or so. During the telogen phase the follicle appears inactive, and the hair shaft may also be shed during this period. Shedding hairs are a normal part of the cycle of hair growth. Shed hairs may appear on bedding, on clothing, in combs and brushes, and many shed hairs simply go down the drain after shampooing. The point is that some hair loss every day is normal.

Anagen Phase

Catagen

Telogen

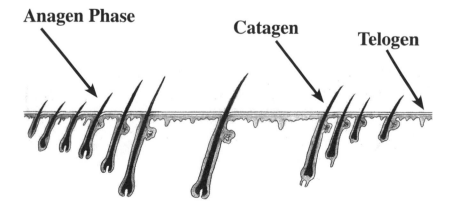

At the end of the telogen phase, the hair follicle enters the anagen phase again and begins to grow back to normal size. A new hair bulb is formed and a new hair shaft begins to grow, and the cycle of hair growth continues.

While many fur-bearing animals have hair follicles with synchronized growth and shedding phases, in humans the growth phase of hair follicles are not normally synchronized with their neighbors. This means that the hair follicles on people's scalps are in different stages of growth, regression, or rest at any given time. But because the anagen (growth) phase lasts much longer than the other phases, the vast majority (ninety percent) of hair follicles on people are in some part of the growth phase, while only a small percentage are in the catagen (regression) or telogen (rest) phase. Growing hairs are not easily shed; however hair follicles in the catagen or telogen phase shed their hairs easily.

On average, young people with a full head of dark-colored hair have about 100,000 hair follicles on their scalp. Redheads often have slightly more than 100,000 scalp hair follicles, while blondes typically have fewer hair follicles. On average, about fifty to100 hair follicles end the anagen phase each day, which is when the follicle begins to loosen its "grip" on the hair shaft, and the hair may be shed. Therefore shedding fifty to100 hairs on any particular day is perfectly normal. Of course, about fifty to100 hair follicles also re-enter the anagen phase each day, and begin growing new hairs as well, but this is less noticeable.

3

The Cause of Most Hair Loss

The most common type of hair loss occurs in a predicable pattern, and pattern hair loss occurs when the normal cycle of hair growth changes. Usually pattern hair loss starts slowly, and continues to get progressively worse. Progressive pattern hair loss is a common occurrence among men, and less apparent but still quite common among women. While men typically suffer pattern baldness with receding hairlines and bald spots on the crown of the head, women typically experience generalized thinning hair over the entire top of the head. And as we age, the occurrence and degree of hair loss increases.

There have been numerous causes blamed for pattern hair loss, including "hot blood," excessive blood circulation in the scalp, inadequate blood circulation in the scalp, wearing hats, brushing the hair too much, brushing too little, dirty scalps, oily scalps, hormones in scalp oil, dandruff, various diseases, excessively tight scalps, inadequate oxygen reaching the hair follicles, inadequate nutrition or nutritional deficiencies, "sleeping" hair follicles, and hairs "stuck" in the hair follicles, to name just some of the "hair loss causes" offered by scientists and charlatans over the years. Chapter 5, "Hair Loss Treatment History," presents a sample of the hundreds of "remedies" that over the years have been offered to those suffering from hair loss. Most of these "cures" are based on "hair loss causes" that simply are not true.

And while it is true that there are many possible reasons for a particular individual's hair loss, including real diseases, certain medications, and even hair loss as a reaction to severe stressful incidents, the vast majority of those suffering progressive hair loss, or pattern baldness, have simply inherited the tendency for hair loss from their parents. The cause of most hair loss is genetics. Almost all pattern hair loss is caused by heredity, from genes passed on by both maternal and paternal ancestors.

Hair loss caused by disease, medication, and stress are discussed in Chapter 4, "Other Hair Loss Causes," and a board certified dermatologist should treat these conditions. A dermatologist is a medical doctor trained specifically to diagnose and treat conditions affecting the hair, skin, and nails. If you suspect that your hair loss is due to something other than genetics, schedule an examination with a dermatologist. Information on selecting a doctor is presented in Chapter 17, "Choosing a Physician."

...the vast majority of those suffering progressive hair loss, or pattern baldness, have simply inherited the tendency for hair loss from their parents. The cause of most hair loss is genetics.

Most people with hair loss simply have a genetic tendency to start losing hair at a certain age, a condition that if untreated will get progressively worse. An understanding of this truth will help you to determine what you can really do about your hair loss.

Almost everyone suffers from a tendency for hair loss to some degree, as very few of us when we are in our fifties, sixties, and seventies will have the hair we had in our teens. The degree of hair loss becomes more apparent as we age. Those individuals with a greater genetic predisposition for hair loss usually start losing their hair earlier and to a greater degree, than those with a lesser genetic predisposition.

By age twenty-five, approximately twenty percent of men will show some signs of hair loss, but by age sixty the percentage will climb to about seventy-five percent. Of the seventy-five percent of men showing signs of hair loss by age sixty, about half these will have significant baldness on the front and top of their heads. Women also

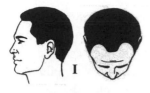

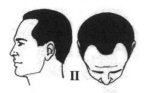

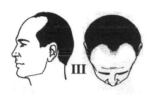

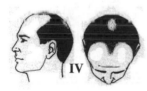

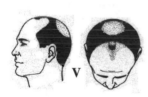

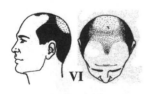

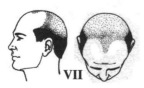

Norwood scale for male pattern hair loss

experience hair thinning as a result of their hair follicle's genetic programming; noticeable hair loss however, in women typically occurs after menopause.

While the entire genetic mechanism that causes hair loss is not completely understood, we do know that in individuals with pattern hair loss, certain hair follicles are genetically programmed to be more sensitive to a hormone circulating in the blood called dihydrotestosterone, commonly abbreviated as DHT. DHT is one of several hormones classified as androgens, often referred to as "male" hormones. DHT is formed from testosterone, the most well known androgen. While men past puberty have higher levels of androgen hormones in their blood than women, it is normal for women to have some androgens, including both testosterone and DHT, circulating in their blood. Just like men with pattern baldness, some women inherit hair follicles with a genetic sensitivity to DHT, which signals pattern hair loss to their DHT-sensitive hair follicles.

The cause of pattern hair loss in both men and women is DHT in the blood signaling hair follicles genetically programmed to be sensitive to DHT to stop growing new hairs.

Hair follicles sensitive to DHT must be exposed to a high enough level of DHT in the blood over a long enough period of time before they get the message to start shutting down. And the message has to continue for years before a hair follicle completely stops producing new hairs. Some hair restoration medications interfere with the conversion of testosterone to DHT reducing the strength of the DHT message, and others block the receptor sites on hair follicle cells so the DHT message does not get through. But even in men and women with a strong inherited tendency for pattern hair loss, there are hair follicles that are not sensitive to DHT, and these follicles continue to grow new hairs for a lifetime.

In men with pattern baldness, the hair follicles that are most sensitive to DHT are generally located at the temples, the hairline, and on the crown of the head. This "pattern" of sensitive hair follicles in men is the reason the condition is commonly called "Male Pattern Baldness."

In women with pattern hair loss, the DHT-sensitive follicles are distributed over a wider area, and the hair loss pattern is less defined. Usually there is generalized thinning over the entire top of the head, with less thinning along the sides and on the back of the head. Women with an inherited tendency for hair loss typically have follicles sensitive to DHT distributed over the tops of their heads.

Normal hair follicles go through a growth cycle (described in the previous chapter) that lasts roughly four to six years, ending with the hair shaft being shed, and a brief resting period after which the

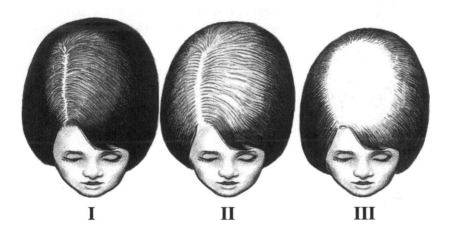

I   II   III

Ludwig Scale for female pattern hair loss

growth cycle starts over again with a new hair beginning to grow from the hair follicle.

But hair follicles that are sensitive to DHT, and that receive the DHT message to shut down, begin to have shorter anagen (growth) phases. The DHT circulating in the blood seems to signal these sensitive hair follicles to stop growing hair before the normal growth phase would have ended. Instead of four to six years, the growth cycle shortens to three to four years, and then one to two years, and eventually the hair follicles affected by DHT simply stop producing new hairs altogether, and stay in a sort of telogen (resting) phase. As the growth phase of the follicles becomes shorter, the hairs grown by those follicles do not grow as long as they once did.

Scalp hairs grow approximately one-half inch per month, which works out to about six inches per year. If the growth phase of a follicle is six years long, the hair grown by that follicle could reach thirty-six inches in length if it were not cut. But if the growth phase shortens to two years, the maximum length of the hair would be only twelve inches. Eventually, as the anagen phase continues to shorten, the hairs produced by the hair follicle may only grow out an inch or less before they are shed.

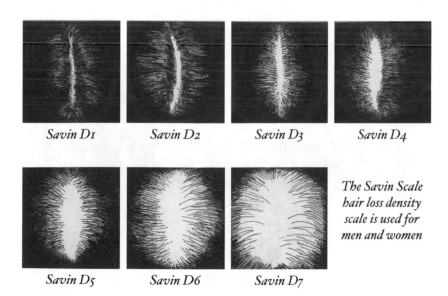

Savin D1   *Savin D2*   *Savin D3*   *Savin D4*

Savin D5   *Savin D6*   *Savin D7*

The Savin Scale hair loss density scale is used for men and women

It is believed that each hair follicle is genetically programmed for a limited number of growth cycles. The shorter the duration of each cycle, the sooner a particular hair follicle goes through all of its growth cycles and stops producing a new hair.

For example, if a particular hair follicle is programmed to have twenty complete growth cycles, each lasting an average of five years, then that hair follicle will continue producing new hairs for 100 years (twenty growth cycles at five years each). But if that hair follicle is sensitive to DHT circulating in the blood, the growth cycles will begin to shorten, and the follicle's twenty-cycle life may only last until age fifty, or forty, or thirty. And some hair follicles are programmed to have fewer than twenty growth cycles, which is why some men start showing frontal hairline recession before age twenty, while other DHT-sensitive follicles continue growing hairs until age thirty or age forty.

But there's more bad news for those who have inherited pattern hair loss. DHT affects sensitive hair follicles in another way as well: it results in thinner and less pigmented strands of hair. Normally, a hair follicle shrinks in size after the anagen (growth) phase, and the hair shaft falls out during the catagen or telogen phase. As the follicle begins a new anagen phase, it grows back to its original size, and it produces a new hair of normal thickness.

There is evidence that hair follicles that are sensitive to DHT do not return to their full size after the telogen phase. In each succes-

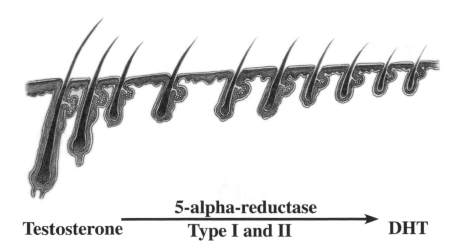

Testosterone $\xrightarrow[\text{Type I and II}]{\text{5-alpha-reductase}}$ DHT

sive growth cycle, the hair follicles become smaller and smaller. This is significant because the hairs produced by these miniaturized hair follicles are themselves thinner and less pigmented than normal hairs. Over time the affected hair follicles only produce nearly transparent "peach fuzz" hairs instead of full size normally colored hairs. And finally they produce no new hairs at all.

So DHT affects sensitive hair follicles two ways: first, it shortens the hair growth cycle, which "ages" the hair follicles. Second, it causes miniaturization of the hair follicles. The result of these two effects are shorter hairs, increasingly finer and less pigmented hairs, and eventually less hair altogether.

But there is still hope for people with pattern hair loss!

First, anybody with partial hair loss can benefit to some degree from careful hair styling, and certain hair care products. And even people with total hair loss can appear to have more hair with the use

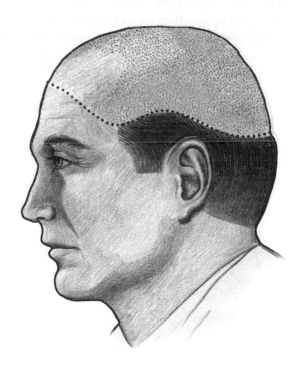

*Hair follicles on the front
and top of the head are sensitive to DHT.*

of a hairpiece or a wig. These cosmetic treatments for hair loss are described in Chapter 7, "Cosmetic Treatments."

Second, there are certain medications that have been proven to be effective at protecting sensitive hair follicles from DHT, and other medications that reduce the amount of testosterone in the blood being converted into DHT, thereby reducing the amount of DHT in the blood. These medications help to slow hair loss, and in some people, they can actually reverse recent hair loss, sometimes quite dramatically. Medications that stop hair loss and may reverse hair loss are described in Chapter 9, "Drugs that Grow Hair."

Third, in most people with inherited pattern hair loss, including both men and women, only the hair follicles on the front and top of the head are sensitive to DHT. The hair follicles on the sides and back of the head are not as much affected by the DHT in the blood. It is these DHT-resistant hair follicles on the back and sides of the head that are moved around to the front and top of the head with hair restoration surgery, thereby creating the appearance of a fuller head of hair. The principles and history of hair restoration surgery are covered in Chapters 10 and 11, and the state-of-the-art transplant procedure called follicular unit micrografting is described in Chapter 12.

4

Other Hair Loss Causes

A wide range of factors other than genetics can result in hair loss, and many of these conditions are temporary and can be effectively treated by a dermatologist. Diffuse non-scarring loss is usually androgenetic alopecia in men and women but can include telogen effluvium, and systemic diseases such as thyroid, iron deficiency, dermatomitis. Patchy scarring loss can be due to follimlites (bacterial infection of the hairs), lichen planilaris and discird lupus. Patchy non-scarring alopecia can be due to ringworm, trichotillomania, traction alopecia, and syphilis. Hair loss causes that are not based on genetics are discussed in this chapter, including the following:

- Autoimmune disorders
- Diseases
- Nutritional deficiencies
- Poisons
- Prescription drugs
- Chemotherapy drugs
- Radiation exposure
- Stress
- Physical trauma to the scalp
- Hair loss following childbirth
- Psychological
- Hair styling techniques
- Hair styling products

Autoimmune Disorders

Autoimmune disease occurs when the body's immune system mistakenly attacks itself. In a fairly common autoimmune disorder called alopecia areata, the white blood cells attack the deepest part of the hair follicle, commonly referred to as the bulb area, resulting in temporary hair loss.

Alopecia areata is probably the second most common cause of hair loss after androgenetic alopecia (inherited predisposition for hair loss). Most people affected by alopecia areata first develop one or two small bald patches on their scalp which persist for several months, after which they eventually re-grow hair in those areas.

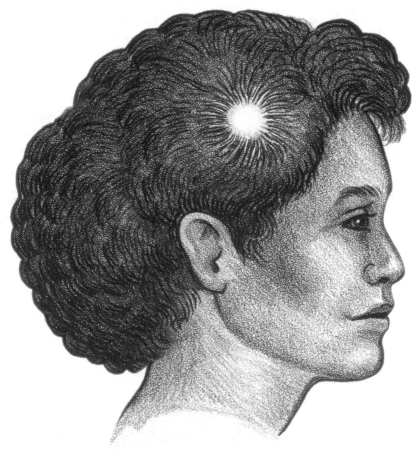

Alopecia areata

Frequently the size and duration of the bald patches increase with subsequent episodes of the disease. Some people with this condition may suffer larger and more persistent bald patches in their very first episode, and some lose all the hair on their scalp, a condition called alopecia totalis. Even more extreme is the loss of all body hair, called alopecia universalis. In some cases the hair loss persists for long durations; nevertheless there is always the possibility of hair regrowth because the inflammation occurs in the bulb area of the hair follicle, which is regenerated with each hair follicle growth cycle.

The National Alopecia Areata Foundation estimates that variations of this condition will affect approximately two percent of the population at some point in their lives, usually beginning during childhood. Hair loss from alopecia areata is not life threatening; however, the bald patches occur suddenly and recur unpredictably causing profound psychological disruptions in the lives of many people affected. The loss of hair due to alopecia areata in children can be psychologically devastating. Treatments with medications such as cortisone injections and minoxidil lotion have limited success.

Treated bald patches may regrow new hair; however new bald patches on other parts of the scalp often occur soon after. Some people with alopecia areata choose to wear their scalp bald, shaving what hair they have. For adults with extensive or total hair loss, there are also cosmetic options such as hats, turbans, scarves, and full-cap wigs that cover the entire scalp. Wigs have several drawbacks as a treatment for young children with alopecia areata. Wigs are fragile and expensive, and can be treated roughly by young children. But more significantly, wigs present a psychological issue for young children in that they suggest that the child is "not OK" as they are. Regardless of whether the affected child chooses to cover their scalp or not, it is beneficial to educate their classmates at school about the condition to temper the inevitable—and usually unwanted—attention that hair loss at a young age attracts.

Another autoimmune disease that can result in hair loss is lupus erythematosus. This autoimmune disease affects the bulge area of the hair follicle rather than the bulb, and can cause permanent hair loss. A dermatologist should treat autoimmune conditions affecting the hair.

OTHER DISEASES

In addition to autoimmune diseases, a wide variety of other disease conditions can cause hair loss.

Fungal infections on the scalp such as ringworm (tinea capitis), kerion, and favus can result in hair loss. Bacterial infections on the scalp such as folliculitis, furuncles, and carbuncles can cause thin hair. Skin cancers—such as metastatic carcinoma and sclerosing basal cell carcinoma—can also cause hair loss.

In rare cases, certain skin diseases such as severe eczema, and lichen planus (which is called lichen planopilaris when it affects the scalp), and psoriasis can result in hair loss. Thyroid and endocrine gland disorders such as hypothyroidism and hypopituitarism can result in thin hair and brittle hair that breaks easily. Leprosy, shingles (herpes zoster infection), and advanced stages of syphilis have all been noted to cause hair loss.

NUTRITIONAL DEFICIENCIES

Nutritional deficiencies are rarely a cause of hair loss despite the marketing of a wide variety of nutritional supplements that claim to somehow enhance hair growth or hair health. Of the possible nutritional deficiencies that can cause thinning hair, iron deficiency anemia is most common, and when it occurs it is more frequently seen in women. Iron deficiency anemia is a result of a decreased amount of red blood cells in the blood because of inadequate iron reserves in the body.

There are several causes for this condition, including inadequate consumption of iron-containing foods, poor absorption of iron in foods or supplements, and loss of blood.

The main sources of iron in a typical western diet include meat, egg yolks, poultry, fish, legumes (lentils, dried peas and beans), whole grains, iron-fortified cereal products and iron-containing multivitamin tablets. Poor absorption of iron can result from disease conditions or from certain medications that interfere with iron absorption. Low red blood cell count from periodic blood loss can contribute to anemia because the body normally recycles the iron in worn out red blood cells. If the blood is lost, the iron in those cells is lost as well.

Menstruation is the most common cause of blood loss-induced iron deficiency anemia; however; blood loss can also result from injury, frequent donation of blood, and internal bleeding from digestive system ulcers and various disease conditions.

The first step in determining if iron deficiency anemia as a cause of a hair loss condition is a blood test for ferritin levels. Ferritin is an iron-storing protein that circulates in the blood and reflects the body's iron reserve level. Just taking an iron supplement is not likely to stop hair loss. If a serum ferritin blood test indicates a deficiency, the next step is to determine the cause of the iron deficiency, and to effectively treat the condition. Many doctors and laboratories assume the normal range of serum ferritin to be 10-230 grams per liter. But in the past few years it has been found that women with levels below seventy have an increased chance of hair loss. Inadequate dietary iron can be treated with iron supplement tablets however, iron absorption problems may require switching medications or injections of iron supplements, and blood loss treatments vary according to the cause.

In addition to iron deficiency anemia, severe "crash" diets, and psychological disorders that result in extreme nutritional imbalances such as anorexia and bulimia, can also result in hair loss. Going without food for several days, or even several weeks, will not cause hair loss. But severe swings in nutrition and body weight from "crash" diets over several months time may begin to affect hair condition.

The American Journal of Clinical Nutrition published a study of two adult hospital patients who were unable to use their intestines to digest food. The patients were fed intravenously a diet that happened to be deficient in the B-complex vitamin biotin. Biotin deficiency is extremely rare because in addition to being present in many types of food, it is also manufactured by the friendly bacteria that live in normal intestines. Because these patients had inactive intestines, their intestinal bacteria did not produce adequate biotin, and they suffered hair loss as a result. When biotin was added to the intravenous diet, hair growth resumed.

With most nutritional deficiency-caused hair loss, hair growth resumes with adequate consumption of the missing nutrient.

POISONS

Certain poisons can cause hair loss when consumed in less than lethal doses. In many cases, hair loss is one of the first signs of poisoning. Warfarin, a common ingredient in commercial rat poisons, can cause hair loss when consumed in large amounts by humans. It is prescribed in smaller amounts for humans as a medicine used for thinning the blood.

Certain metal salts and heavy metals including arsenic, mercury, bismuth, lithium, thallium, cadmium, and gold are poisonous, and can cause hair loss as a result of prolonged inhalation in industrial environments or by ingestion. Organic forms of metal salts tend to be more readily absorbed and more slowly eliminated, and are more toxic. Arsenic is used in glass manufacturing, metal refining, silicon chip manufacturing, insecticides, rat poisons, fungicides, and wood preservatives. Arsenic poisoning has resulted from ingestion, and also from inhaling fumes from arsenic-preserved wood intended for outdoor use. Mercury poisoning has resulted from consumption of mercury-containing seafood and also from exposure to mercury-containing medications, paint, fungicides and industrial products. Prior to 1972, thallium sulfate was a common ingredient in pesticides and rat poisons, and poisoning from accidental ingestion by children was often discovered as a result of their hair loss. Consumption of 50,000 to 250,000 Units of vitamin A daily over many months can cause hair loss. Boric acid, a common household pesticide, can cause hair loss when consumed over a period of time.

PRESCRIPTION DRUGS

There are many categories of prescription drugs that present a risk of temporary hair loss as a possible side effect. Chemotherapy drug treatment almost always causes hair loss because the drugs target rapidly dividing cells typical of cancer. See Chapter 8 and Appendix 2 for a complete discussion.

RADIATION EXPOSURE

Ionizing radiation such as the type used for cancer treatment, also affects rapidly dividing cells most severely, and, as a result of exposure to radiation, actively producing hair follicles are shut down. The amount of hair loss from radiation exposure varies, however.

With radiation treatment, only hair that is in the treatment field is affected. When the treatment field includes the scalp, hair loss generally begins about two to three weeks after the first radiation treatment. Usually the hair begins to grow back three to four months after the last treatment; however, with high doses of radiation, there is a risk of permanent hair loss in the treatment area.

STRESS

Stress can cause a type of hair loss called telogen effluvium. This condition is not caused by the general accumulated stress of ordinary interactions with people at home and at work, but rather by sudden severe emotional or physiological incidents. Severe stressful events can cause some or most actively growing hair follicles to prematurely shift into the regression phase, and then the resting phase, during which the hairs fall out easily.

There is usually a delay of a few weeks to a few months before the shedding is noticeable, but after this delay the shedding seems to occur quite suddenly. Because the shedding is delayed, this type of hair loss is often a mystery to the person suffering the condition. The stressful event that triggered it is frequently forgotten, and it is rarely thought to be connected with the "new problem."

Examples of sudden severe emotionally stressful events include the death or terminal illness of a family member or close friend, marriage, divorce, and unexpected job loss. Severe physiological stressful events shock the body, and some examples are heart attacks, major surgery, and illnesses with prolonged high fever such as malaria, viral pneumonia, and severe cases of the flu.

In most cases of telogen effluvium, the hair follicles recover and soon shift back to the regular growth cycle.

However, repeated instances of telogen effluvium can result in premature hair loss in people predisposed to lose their hair late in life. The average growth cycle of a hair follicle takes about five years, but each follicle is "genetically programmed" for only a limited number of growth cycles. For example, if a particular hair follicle were "genetically programmed" for only ten growth cycles, after about fifty years that follicle would stop producing new hairs. When all the follicles at the hairline or crown of the head are "genetically programmed" this way, a receding hairline or bald spot appears after all the growth cycles for the follicles in those areas have been cycled through.

Each incidence of telogen effluvium uses up one "life" of the affected hair follicles. So instead of having a receding hairline or bald spot at age fifty, the hair loss may occur a few years earlier. This is not a significant issue if telogen effluvium occurs once or twice in a lifetime; however, accelerated hair loss can result from repeated severe stressful events, if each instance triggers a new round of telogen effluvium.

I had a patient who was totally bald when I met him at age seventy, and he had lost all his hair by age twenty-two. He had worked on the Panama Canal fifty years earlier, and for two straight years starting when he was twenty he suffered repeated bouts of severe fever from episodes of malaria. Each time he suffered from malaria induced fever he experienced telogen effluvium, lost what hair he had, and his hair follicles lost another "life." After ten or fifteen malaria stress cycles, at the age of twenty-two, he had the hair he would have had at age seventy. Which unfortunately for him was no hair at all.

Physical Trauma to the Scalp

Physical trauma to the scalp, such as from wounds from accidental cutting or impact, thermal burns from heat or fire, chemical burns from acids, alkalis, or other caustic substances, and from freezing due to exposure to severe cold or liquefied gas such as liquid nitrogen can cause permanent hair loss. Continuous pressure on the scalp from a tight fitting helmet or other headgear worn every day can in some people cause permanent hair loss. Hair loss due to a tight fitting helmet will cause loss only at the site of too much pressure and is a result of friction and pressure breaking the hair shafts. This will not cause permanent baldness unless prolonged pressure prevents blood from getting to the hairs. Newborn babies sometimes have a one-inch bald spot on the side of the head from prolonged pressure against the side of their mother's pelvis. Lastly, trauma injuries can be the result of elective cosmetic surgery, such as from synthetic fiber implants, improperly performed hair transplants, or radical scalp lifts that result in scalp tissue death.

Usually there are only two types of treatment for physical trauma to the scalp. One is surgery: Either cutting out the injured area by performing a scalp reduction procedure, or by placing hair transplant grafts into the scar tissue at the injured area. The second option is a hairpiece or full cap wig.

Hair Loss Following Childbirth

Childbirth often causes a temporary form of hair loss called post-partum telogen effluvium. During the second and third trimester of pregnancy, hair follicles on many women remain in the active growing phase, rather than enter the resting and shedding phases, as they normally would have.

During pregnancy this results in a higher proportion of actively growing hair follicles, and thicker more luxuriant hair. However, within one to three months following childbirth, the hair follicles go back to their regular growth cycle. All the follicles that would have been resting and shedding over the previous six months or so stop growing all at the same time, and a larger than usual amount of hair is shed.

Discontinuation of some birth control pills can also result in hair shedding, because some oral contraceptives mimic to some degree the hormonal effects of pregnancy. The condition is temporary, but can be disturbing to new mothers, who already have their hands full taking care of a new baby.

Psychological

A somewhat mysterious type of hair loss results from compulsive hair pulling, a psychological condition called trichotillomania. Young children may exhibit this behavior in response to anxiety. Counseling to address the issues causing anxiety is the best long-term treatment; however cutting the hair short to make pulling more difficult may also help in the short term.

Hair Styling Techniques

A type of hair loss called traction alopecia can result from certain hair-styling techniques that pull tightly on the hairs, such as tight "cornrow" braids and pigtails. Modifying these styling techniques so that they are not too tight solves the problem.

Cosmetic products and procedures that weaken or damage the hair shaft can result in hair loss. For example, highly alkaline hair relaxers and straighteners, as well as acidic permanent wave treatments, can cause hair loss. Hair bleaching and coloring agents, when used excessively, can weaken the hair shaft and result in breakage and hair loss. Hair growth resumes after the products are discontinued.

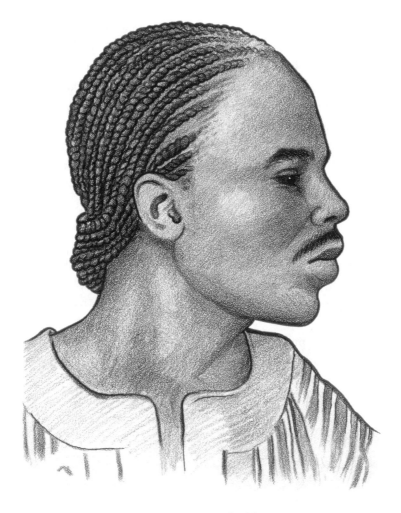

Cornrow braids

5

Hair Loss Treatment History

Since the beginning of recorded history, men and women have searched out cures for hair loss. Over the last 5,000 years, there have been many cosmetic treatments that give the illusion of more hair, a few medical treatments that use drugs to affect the hair follicles, and some surgical treatments that remove bald areas or move hair follicles around. And these are just the treatments that work.

Countless herbal solutions, medical-sounding cosmetics, nutritional supplements, pills, oils, lotions, and shampoos have been advanced, with little or no result. Electric shock devices, ultraviolet light-emitting instruments, LED, laser, and vacuum-cap machines have all been alleged to help stimulate the follicles to grow hair. Even spiritual solutions have been advanced. In fact, prayer may indeed be a better solution than most of the treatments that follow.

What is noteworthy about the history of hair loss treatment is this: despite real advances in genuinely effective cosmetics, medical treatments, and surgical procedures, bogus hair loss solutions continue to be marketed today with astonishing success. Their sales are astonishing, that is. Despite their wild claims, most of the products marketed as hair loss solutions don't have a scientifically measurable positive effect. In other words, they don't stop hair loss or grow new hair. But people are so concerned about hair loss, they want to believe some "miracle cure" will work for them.

3000 BC

Wigs and hairpieces of various sorts were popular among upper class Assyrians, Sumerians, Cretans, Carthaginians, Persians, and Greeks in the Fertile Crescent area of the Middle East. Around this same time period, a compendium of medical knowledge that included prescriptions for hair loss treatment was passed on from generation to generation among Fertile Crescent area healers.

1553 BC

The Ebers Papyrus, discovered in Luxor, Egypt, is believed to include medical

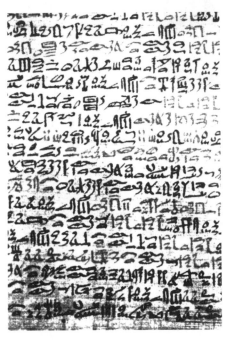

A portion of the Ebers Papyrus the first prescription for hair loss

information drawn from the earlier described compendium of medical knowledge which was collected 2,000 years earlier. The Ebers Papyrus is the oldest complete medical text ever found, and it is devoted to treatments for various skin diseases and cosmetic conditions. It includes the oldest known written prescription for treating baldness: a mixture of iron oxide, red lead, onions, alabaster, honey and fat from a variety of animals including snakes, crocodiles, hippopotamuses and lions. The mixture was to be swallowed, after first reciting a magical invocation to the Sun God:

This is a prescription for hair restoration from the Ebers Papyrus

"O Shining one, thou who hoverest above!

O Xare! O Disk of the Sun!

O Protector of the Divine Neb-Apt!"

1500 BC

Wigs were popular among Egyptian royalty at this time as well, and a number of elaborate and well-preserved hairpieces have been found in tombs by archaeologists. Many Egyptian wigs were ornate creations constructed of linen fiber as well as human hair, while others made of metal were more helmet-like. As an example of the importance hair played in certain cultures, certain Egyptian royalty also used "facial hair wigs," specifically fake beards, to signify power. Both male and female royalty wore the fake beards.

420 BC

In ancient Greece, Hippocrates, the Father of Modern Medicine, tried many medical solutions for his own progressive hair loss, and he was the first to describe an effective surgical solution to hair loss. One of his medical formulas was a mixture of opium, horseradish, pigeon droppings, beetroot, and various spices that were applied to the head. It didn't work. Hippocrates eventually became so bald that two thousand years later, we refer to extreme cases of hair loss as "Hippocratic baldness."

Hippocrates recorded the first surgical solution to baldness. In his collection of astute observations called the "Aphorisms of Hippocrates," he noted that Persian Army eunuchs guarding the king's harem never experienced hair loss. He noticed that virile "hot blooded" men went bald, but since eunuchs were castrated, they lacked "hot blood," and therefore retained their hair. In Aphorism XXVIII he states: "Eunuchs are not affected by gout, nor do they become

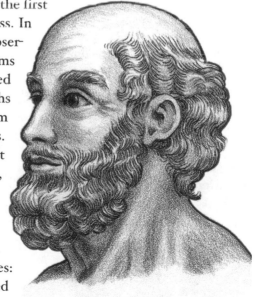

Hippocrates

37

bald." We now know that it is true that castration before or shortly after puberty reduces testosterone and DHT levels in the blood to such a degree that genetic hair loss is prevented.

Approximately 2,400 years later, in March 1995, researchers at Duke University finally published the same results. The Duke University researchers concluded: "While castration may be a cure, it is not commercially acceptable," (reprinted from The *San Francisco Chronicle*). The search for hair loss cures went on.

44 BC

In ancient Rome, hair continued to be a symbol of power and virility. This presented a problem for Julius Caesar, whose hairline was receding even as his empire was expanding. He developed some cosmetic solutions to his hair loss problem. First he began growing it long in the back and combing it straight forward over his bald spot. Sort of a "comb forward" instead of a "comb over." This didn't seem to work all that well, perhaps because hair gel would not be invented for another 2,000 years. So Caesar then took to wearing a laurel wreath around his head to hide his hair loss. The trademark wreath soon became a symbol of power and virility.

1624

Over 1,600 years later, King Louis XIII of France began wearing a full wig to camouflage his thinning hair. Soon, other members of the court followed his example, regardless of their own hair condition. Wigs became symbols of power. The height, length, and bulk of wigs increased with each

Nobility wearing wigs

decade, and giant powdered wigs soon became the fashion in all French courts.

1660

In England, King Charles II was restored to the throne after his exile in Versailles where he had been exposed to the French wig craze. The English were not to be outdone by the French. Within a short time, more elaborate giant powdered wigs were worn in English courts than had ever appeared in France.

1700S

Upper class American colonists picked up the wig fashion, and by the late 18th century most wealthy people wore false hair to signify their elevated class. However, the American War of Independence and the subsequent French Revolution caused the look of royalty and elevated class distinction to fall out of favor, and wigs pretty much disappeared from the scene.

1800S

This was the heyday of the "snake oil" salesmen, and for the next hundred years bottles of hair loss cures with names like "Mrs. Allen's World Hair Restorer," "Ayers Hair Vigour," "East India Oil Hair Restoration," "Skookum Root Hair Growth," "Westphall Auxiliator," "Imperial Hair Regenerator" and the ever popular "Barry's Tricopherous" were sold to hopeful buyers seeking a cure for their hair loss from "modern medicine."

A hundred years later, "snake oil" cures for hair loss continue to be marketed, except now they're sold by beauty salons and barber shops, by mail, cable television, over the Internet, and with great success to listeners of talk radio programs. The names of the products have changed to things like Helsinki Formula, Foliplexx, Revivogen, Nioxin, Kevis, and Fabao to name just a few. The same outlandish performance promises fool vulnerable consumers.

Amazingly enough, Barry's Tricopherous, which was founded in 1801, was still being sold in Central America as late as the 1970s when a bottle was discovered for sale in a Honduras pharmacy. It is now part of my collection of bogus hair loss remedies. The label states: "Guarantees to Restore the Hair to Bald Heads and to Make it Grow Thick, Long and Soft." The bottle contains alcohol, water, and coloring.

1850S

During the Victorian era in England, a popular hair loss treatment was cold India tea applied to the scalp, followed by a vigorous rubbing of the balding area with fresh lemon juice. This hair loss treatment would probably be better to sip on a hot day than apply to the scalp. It didn't grow hair.

1900S

The wearing of hats by nearly all men in urban areas around this time was blamed for causing hair loss. Anti-hat advocates urged men to let their hair follicles "breathe" and to allow their scalps to enjoy the benefits of "sun baths" and "air baths." No one seemed to notice the countless men who wore hats who did not lose their hair.

1905

Allied Merke Thermocap

The industrial age brought new inventions to the marketplace, solving a countless number of life's little problems. In St. Louis, the Evans Vacuum Cap Company marketed a suction device that: "...exercises the scalp and helps to circulate stagnant blood, feeding the shrunken hair roots, and causing the hair to grow..."

1920S

People still suffered from hair loss, and modern science continued to work on this problem. Devices using the miracle of electricity started to replace mechanical hair restoration machines. In the United States, exotic gas-filled clear glass combs with names like "Master Violet Ray" and "Super Marvel" glowed with purple light as they generated an electric charge. The electrified comb was raked across the scalp to stimulate hair growth. Amazingly, some of these devices continued to be sold until the 1950s.

1922

In his book, *Hair Culture*, health advocate Bernarr MacFadden wrote: "There is more quackery rampant in connection with hair and scalp care—both by the medical profession and by drug and lotion manufacturers—than there is in any other specialty ever devised for the exploitation of ailing humans." He then went on to say that most hair loss is caused by lack of physical vigor and unhygienic scalp conditions. He prescribed scalp massage, hair pulling, and vigorous brushing of the scalp.

1925

The Allied Merke Institute in New York City began selling the Thermocap Treatment device, claiming to stimulate circulation, cleanse clogged-up pores, and nourish dormant hair bulbs

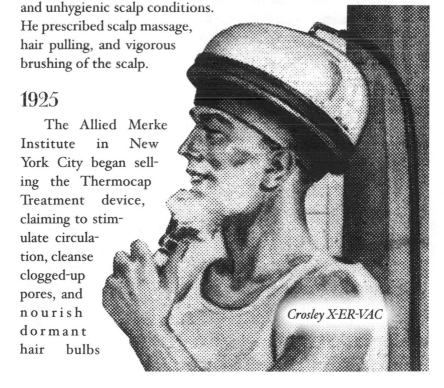

Crosley X-ER-VAC

with heat and blue light from a special actinic quartz ray bulb. The quartz ray treatment took only fifteen minutes a day. Along with the Thermocap device, the complete Treatment included the Merke Tonic, Merke Dandruff Treatment, and Merke Shampoo Cream.

1936

In Cincinnati, the Crosley Radio Corporation diversified a bit from radios, and offered an electric scalp vacuum device claimed to be a "Therapeutic Method for Hair Growth" and called it the X-ER-VAC. It was available for home, local clinic, barbershop, and beauty shop use.

1939

In Japan, dermatologist Dr. Shoji Okuda, published in the October issue of the Japanese *Journal of Dermatology* his method for using hair transplant grafts to replace hair lost from the scalp, eyebrow, mustache, and pubic hair areas. This was the first published account of the modern hair transplantation technique, and it worked! Dr. Okuda removed hair follicles from the back of his patient's heads, and transplanted the grafts to new locations to give the look of having more hair. His work went largely unnoticed in the West because of World War II.

1952

Dr. Norman Orentreich, a dermatologist in New York City, was doing a study on vitiligo, a skin pigment disorder. His study involved transferring patches of skin from one part of a patient's body to another. It was noted that a skin graft taken from a hair bearing area, when placed in a non-hair bearing area, continued to grow hair at the new site. Soon after making this observation, Dr. Orentreich placed ten punch grafts bearing hair on the front part of the scalp of a patient with severe frontal hair loss. The grafts continued to grow hair in the new location. Dr. Orentreich reported the successful results of the first hair transplant procedure performed in the United States in a paper submitted to the *Archives of Dermatology*. The reviewers of that journal said the reported results "were not possible" and rejected the paper.

1959

Dr. Norman Orentreich was finally able to publish his "donor dominance" theory in the New York Academy of Sciences Journal, popularizing and refining the full size graft hair transplantation technique. The basis of his theory was that plugs of hair follicles taken from the back of the scalp would grow when moved to the front or top of the scalp because those hair follicles were genetically programmed to keep growing hair. It was the particular hair follicles that mattered, not the location on the head. This concept became the foundation for the entire field of hair restoration surgery. For the next twenty years, full-size grafts were the standard technique for hair transplants.

1960S

Despite scientific evidence that genetics was the cause of pattern hair loss, other theories continued to be presented by people whose hair loss solution happened to cure the particular theorized cause. Scalp tightness, for example, was advanced as the reason for hair loss, and surgical procedures to "loosen the scalp" with incisions were performed.

LATE 1960S

The miracle of modified acrylic fiber allowed mass-produced wigs that had the look of human hair to be constructed by machine and sold inexpensively. Soon a whole range of wigs, hairpieces, and other "hair supplements" were introduced, and they were even sold at Tupperware-style "wig parties" in suburban areas.

1968

At age twenty-seven, Sy Sperling got his first hairpiece. He was so thrilled with the success of his new look that concealed a receding hairline, he decided to make non-surgical hair replacements his career. He created Hair Club for Men, marketing "weaves" which were hairpieces attached to the naturally growing hairs around the edges of the bald area. Hair Club for Men grew to become the largest hair replacement company in the world, establishing a research department to make improvements to non-surgical hair appliances.

1969

In the United States, I began my residency training with Dr. James Burks, one of the first doctors to perform hair transplants on a regular basis in the United States. During my residency, I performed hair transplantation procedures every week for three years.

1970S

The "Bald is Beautiful" movement enjoys a brief moment in the spotlight. Bald actors and celebrities such as Yul Brynner and Telly Savalas, appear on TV and in movies with completely bald heads, a concept almost unheard of previously.

1976

Since the 1920s, skin tumors and injured areas of the scalp were removed surgically using a procedure called a "scalp reduction." In this procedure, the damaged tissue was cut out and the edges of the surgical wound were carefully sewn back together in a manner that left only a very small scar. In 1976, doctors Martin Unger and Walter Unger submitted for publication to the *Journal of Plastic and Reconstructive Surgery* an article titled "The Management of Alopecia of the Scalp by a Combination of Excisions and Transplantation." The article described a method of removing healthy, but hairless, scalp tissue from a patient to simultaneously lift up the fringe of permanent growing hair along the sides and back of the head, while making the bald area needing transplants smaller. The article was rejected as "representing nothing new." However, alopecia reductions (bald scalp reductions) soon were regularly performed along with full-size graft hair transplant procedures, because they allowed for increased hair density with full-size graft procedures.

1978

In the United States, for the first time in 5,000 years, a medication has been scientifically proven to reduce the rate of thinning hair and help grow back hairs that have been lost. Minoxidil, a medication taken in pill form for treating severe high blood pressure, was discovered to have this beneficial "side-effect" in some patients.

Clinical trials were established to prove to the U.S. Food and Drug Administration the safety and effectiveness of this promising hair loss treatment medication, but it will be years before the manufacturer can advertise it as a treatment for hair loss. In the meantime, I developed a topical formula containing minoxidil that I applied to my own scalp and prescribed for certain patients.

1979

In San Francisco, I initiated complaints to the FDA, FTC, and California Department of Consumer Affairs against artificial hair implant "clinics," where synthetic fibers were surgically placed into the scalp tissue of "patients." The "patients" at these "clinics" were hoping for a permanent solution to their hair loss, but instead every customer suffered massive scalp inflammation, which often required surgical removal of the affected area, leaving them with unsightly scars as well as less hair. Initially, there was no response from the government agencies, and one bureaucrat even accused me of trying to "stifle competition". Frustrated with government agencies, I went to the news media. The San Francisco Chronicle sent a reporter to the clinic "under cover." The resulting expose revealed that the clinic's "doctor" had no medical license. Criminal charges were filed and the clinic closed. Soon after this incident, artificial hair implants became illegal in California. Five years later, the FDA would ban artificial hair implantation in all states.

1979

Drawing attention to the significance of hair, bald-headed female celebrities begin to appear in the media, including and actress Sigourney Weaver in the movie Alien (1979), and later, singer Sinead O'Connor on her album The Lion and The Cobra (1988).

1980S

In the field of hair transplant surgery, full-size grafts ("plugs") are replaced first by minigrafts and then soon after by micrografts. The new technique of micrografting allows patients to avoid the "under construction" look, and achieves a more natural overall result than most full-size graft procedures.

1984

The United States Food and Drug Administration (FDA) bans synthetic fiber implants, a type of surgical hair restoration procedure where thousands of strands of fibers were implanted in the scalp to simulate the look of real hair. Although the fibers were similar to surgical sutures used by doctors to stitch up wounds, within a short period of time they would cause bumps, inflammation, infection, scars, and even more hair loss.

1988

Minoxidil lotion is the first medication approved by the FDA for treating hair loss. It is sold by prescription only in a two percent solution under the brand name Rogaine.

1988

Dr. Bob Limmer, a dermatologist and hair restoration surgeon practicing in Texas, has his surgical team use stereo microscopes rather than less powerful magnifying glasses while preparing micrografts. The more powerful magnification helps his team to preserve naturally occurring clusters of hair follicles in the donor tissue. This advance in micrografting reduces cutting and the risk of graft failure, while producing grafts that grow more naturally than arbitrarily cut single-hair, two-hair, and three-hair grafts. In 1991, Dr. Limmer publishes an article in Hair Transplant Forum International describing what would become known as follicular unit micrografting.

1989

The FDA restricts all non-prescription hair creams, lotions, and cosmetic products from making medical claims that they can grow hair or prevent baldness. Manufacturers respond by altering their advertising slightly to make medical-sounding claims without actually stating that the products can grow hair.

1990

Another generic medication called finasteride is shown to reverse hair loss, and it is even more effective than minoxidil in preventing baldness. The U.S. FDA originally approved finasteride as a treatment for enlarged prostate glands. New clinical trials begin to test this medication's safety and effectiveness as a hair restoration treatment.

1990S

More bald-headed male celebrities are seen in the media, including basketball superstar Michael Jordan, and Star Trek Next Generation's Captain Picard, portrayed by actor Patrick Stewart.

1991

Hair Club for Men introduces a unique method of eliminating hairpiece "weaves," by using an adhesive to attach the hair appliances directly to the scalp. Glued-on hairpieces soon become the industry standard.

1993

The electric shock method of "awakening" hair follicles never seems to go away. This time a Canadian company called Current Technology Corporation develops a machine that uses low-level electric shocks to treat bald heads. They call the therapy ElectroTrichoGenesis. This electroshock treatment has not been proven to work any better than the electric comb of 1920

1994

In San Francisco, I start taking a low dose of finasteride once a day to preserve my own hair.

1995

In an attempt to simultaneously solve the artificial hair appliance problems of secure attachment and easy removal for hygiene, Dr. Anthony Pignataro, a New York cosmetic surgeon, develops the snap-on hairpiece. In the first part of this new method of hairpiece attachment, surgical-quality titanium sockets are screwed through the scalp into the skull and allowed to fuse with the bone over a period of three months. Then, small gold-alloy snaps are screwed into the sockets. The snaps mate securely with attachments formed into the underside of a custom-made hairpiece. I advised my patients to avoid this procedure due to the risk of a life threatening infection. Osteomyelitis (bone infection) of the skull and retrograde infection into the brain are real possibilities with this procedure.

1995

The FDA approves two percent Rogaine lotion as an over-the-counter drug, meaning it can now be sold without a prescription. Generic versions of minoxidil lotion become available in concentrations up to five percent, and are sold in supermarkets and drugstores.

1995

In the United States, micrografting evolves into Follicular Unit Micrografting and becomes the new state-of-the-art method of hair transplantation. The key to this technique is to identify and preserve the natural clusters of hair follicles from strips of donor tissue, minimizing cutting and risk of damage to the limited supply of donor follicles. In addition, the grafts are kept chilled and moist during all stages of the procedure to further reduce graft failure. I develop several improvements to instrumentation used in Follicular Unit Micrografting, including using cool fluorescent transillumination and a disposable clear vinyl cutting surface with stereomicroscopes during graft preparation.

1995

I am astonished to see artificial fiber implant procedures again advertised as the ultimate solution to hair loss by Ivari International in national magazines such as *Harper's Bazaar.* Their innovation—called the Intra Dermic Micropoint—is a supposed improvement over the knotted fibers used in the past. The innovation appears to be some sort of bead that is surgically implanted into the scalp to anchor each implanted hair. The procedure is illegal in the United States because of severe immune response reactions, so patients who visit the Beverly Hills or New York City clinics of Ivari International are flown to Paris for treatment. The cost of the procedure starts at $60,000.

I immediately contacted the Attorney General's office and filed another complaint. Included in the complaint was a copy of the

February 3, 1979 San Francisco Chronicle article in which I was quoted as follows: "Whether they use real hair, synthetic fibers, and stick it straight in or knot it, it just can't work. There is no known substance that can go through the skin and remain there that won't allow bacteria to migrate down and cause an infection."

1998

Finasteride becomes the second prescription medication approved by the FDA as a hair loss treatment. It is sold in pill form under the brand name Propecia. This medication now makes it possible for men in the early stages of hair loss to keep the hair they have, and even gain back some hair that was recently lost. Eighty-five percent of men stop losing their hair while taking Propecia.

1998

In Canada, a company markets a laser-light treatment that promises to stop hair loss and stimulate hair. With just two thirty-minute sessions twice-weekly, along with regular use of their own branded shower head filter, shampoo, conditioner, and nutritional supplements, they claim that seventeen of eighteen patients in their study showed absolutely no further signs of hair loss, and fifteen of eighteen people showed signs of new hair growth.

2002

A Portland, Oregon firm offers balding men and women the service of storing samples of their hair in a basement room for an annual fee, in the hopes that in the future a cure for baldness will require a hair sample. A staff writer for the *San Francisco Chronicle* interviewed Dr. Alexa Bower Kimball, a dermatologist at the Stanford University Medical Center, and asked if she could think of any reason why someone should bank a sample of his or her hair. Her answer: "Not off the top of my head."

2000-2005

Hair cloning (culturing stem cells from the patient's hair follicle, stem cell transplants, hair multiplication and scalp impregnation therapy are all terms for harvesting hair stem cells for the purpose of transplanting an endless supply of new hairs. All these techniques have been improved upon in the past five years and some doctors have offered potential patients the opportunity of being on a "waiting list" for the procedure when it is approved. Gene therapy to correct androgenetic alopecia has been found to be possible, but it will take years of experience before it will be safe to use on the public. More on this in Chapter 18: Future Hair Loss Treatments.

TODAY

Currently, the most effective cosmetic treatments for hair loss are wigs and hairpieces, which work regardless of the cause of the hair loss. The most effective medicines for androgenetic alopecia (hereditary pattern hair loss) are Propecia for men, and a combination of spironolactone and hormone therapy for women. The most effective surgical procedure for pattern baldness is follicular unit micrografting.

6

Bogus Treatments

Intelligent men and women will buy bogus hair growth treatments. These are treatments that do not work. Despite the claims made in print and television advertisements, on product labels, or by salespeople, most hair growth products do not grow hair. It is amazing to me that people who know better than to believe advertisements for products promising "easy weight loss without dieting," or "face-lifts without surgery," will often give ineffective hair loss treatments a try.

Advertisers for hair restoration products play on their prospect's hopes and fears. Marketers of fake hair loss products often present their own (phony) reasons for hair loss, and then offer their special product that neatly solves the stated cause of the loss. Or they state the actual causes of hair loss, and then claim that their product somehow corrects the problem. People desperately want to believe these useless products work.

Bogus products for treating hair loss cost hopeful consumers millions of dollars each year. They also confuse consumers and distract them from trying hair restoration treatments that really do work.

In the United States, medicines and medical devices that actually affect the function of the body are regulated by the Food and Drug Administration, and are extensively tested in lengthy and expensive clinical trials to assure safety and effectiveness.

To avoid regulation that would show that these products do not work, bogus products claim to the FDA to be either cosmetics having no effect on the body's function, or they claim to be food supplements containing naturally occurring herbal, botanical, vitamin, and enzyme ingredients. Cosmetics and food supplements are more loosely regulated than medicines and medical devices.

But the labeling, and especially the advertising for these products, suggests that they have "medical" properties that somehow stop hair loss or grow new hair. The wording in their advertising is very carefully crafted to sound medically beneficial, but without stepping over the bounds of what the FDA would consider to be a medical claim. They may claim their product "opens the nutrient pathways" or "increases cellular activity" or other such nonsense. And almost always they will claim to have "all natural ingredients with no know side effects."

If a hair restoration treatment sounds too good to be true, it probably is. Before you purchase a treatment for hair loss, consult with a dermatologist and get the facts.

Bogus treatments for hair loss tend to be offered for sale by companies with scientific sounding names, or by "research labs." They are sold by mail-order ads in company-owned health journals, on Internet web sites, on cable TV infomercials, and especially on talk radio advertisements. Multi-level marketing and hair salons are also favorite ways to sell, because another individual (who earns a commission) can make a direct verbal sales pitch explaining that the bogus products "really work."

For example, one product released by a New York firm consists of a three-part "hair care system" that claims to restore hair in nearly all balding men and women. It consists of a DHT blocker, a topical solution and a scalp detoxifying shampoo. The product purportedly treats androgenic alopecia, an inherited condition common in both men and women. Product adds talk about dihydrotestosterone (DHT), the substance largely responsible for shrinking hair follicles that lead to baldness. The product claims to block the effect of DHT on hair follicles, but the label uses obscure and misspelled names of common herbs, only one of which—saw palmetto—has been shown to have any effect on the production of DHT. And the label gives no indication how much saw palmetto the product contains. The scalp lotion included in the three-part system contains minoxidil, an FDA approved hair-loss drug (brand name, Rogaine) now sold over the counter at about ten to twenty dollars for a one-month supply. Minoxidil may help some people grow hair, but the success rate is far below the ninety percent claimed by advertisements. Bottom line: this product, which was a top seller on the internet in early 2004, is a very expensive way to buy an undetermined amount of minoxidil.

In addition to offering a whole series of impressive sounding "solutions" to a wide array of phony hair loss "causes," the sales material for bogus products follow up with "testimonials" from individuals, and sometimes even medical professionals. There is no way to verify these testimonials. Even if verified, there is no way to determine if the "miracle cures" were actually caused by the product being promoted, because there was no scientifically controlled clinical trial. Many types of hair loss are temporary, and hair growth resumes all by itself.

One thing many bogus products have going for them is the placebo effect. When Rogaine was studied, sixteen percent of the placebo group had measurable new hair growth. That's four out of twenty-five people whose state of mind alone brought about real, measurable results. The power of the human mind is enormous.

Think about the economics of an effective hair loss treatment for a moment. Hair loss affects a huge proportion of the world's population, and hundreds of millions of dollars are spent on hair loss treatment every year. A universally effective hair restoration treatment with no side effects would be worth hundreds of millions of dollars a year all by itself. When it would be discovered, it would be on the front page of every newspaper and magazine, and would be featured on every TV and cable show. There would be no need to advertise it on morning talk radio shows or in direct mail pieces.

The following page shows an example of a product costing far more than, and no more effective than, standard treatments.

National Council Against Health Fraud

Enhancing Freedom of Choice through Reliable Health Information   Send This Page

Consumer Health Digest #03-17

Your Weekly Update of News and Reviews
April 29, 2003

Consumer Health Digest is a free weekly e-mail newsletter edited by Stephen Barrett, M.D., and cosponsored by NCAHF and Quackwatch. It summarizes scientific reports; legislative developments; enforcement actions; news reports; Web site evaluations; recommended and nonrecommended books; and other information relevant to consumer protection and consumer decision-making.

FDA warns Avacor marketer. The U.S. Food and Drug Administration has warned Global Vision Products, Inc., that it cannot legally market its Avacor™ Hair Care System without FDA approval. The system includes a "detoxifying shampoo"; a topical formula; and capsules of an herbal "DHT blocker" claimed to "combat the bad chemicals in our body that causes thinning and balding." The topical formula has contained minoxidil, the active ingredient in the approved drug Rogaine. The FDA's etter notes that the presence of minoxidil and the nature of the manufacturer's claims make the components "new drugs" that require proof of safety and effectiveness before marketing. [Woyshner JG. Letter to Anthony Imbroglio, April 2, 2003] Ads for the product have claimed that the capsules work by blocking the follicle-shrinking effect of dihydrotestosterone (DHT), a hormone made from testosterone. The *UC Berkeley Wellness Letter* is skeptical about the capsules and has warned that although minoxidil may help some people grow a little hair, its success rate is far less than the 90% claimed for Avacor. Moreover, nonprescription Rogaine costs much less. [Avacor. UC Berkeley Wellness Letter, March 2003] The doctor featured in Avacor infomercials (David L. Gordon, M.D.) lost his medical license in 1995 after being convicted of defrauding Medicaid. [Gifford B. There's a price on your head. Men's Health, Sept 2002] Global Vision's Web site does not identify minoxidil as an ingredient.

An Online Warning About a Product of Dubious Value

7

Cosmetic Treatments

Cosmetic treatments for hair loss only affect the user's appearance, and not the structure or function of the living cells that make up the body. Cosmetic hair loss treatments are temporary solutions that need to be performed again and again on a regular basis. And cosmetic treatments are reversible, although some treatments such as cutting the hair or shaving the head will take some time to return to the original condition.

HAIR STYLING

A good haircut can go a long way towards improving the appearance of a person with hair loss. It is important to have the right cut for the shape of your head, and for the desired look you are trying to achieve. Hair styling for people with hair loss can either use the existing hair to more effectively camouflage the hair loss, or can involve cutting the hair shorter so that the thin hair is not as apparent.

Using existing hair to camouflage hair loss generally works only when the hair loss area is small, and when there is plenty of existing hair to work with. Comb-overs are not an effective solution, and usually draw more attention to the balding scalp.

Permanent waves, commonly called "perms," are a method of increasing the curliness of existing hair by wrapping strands of hair around rods while treating the hair with chemicals. After a short period of time, the chemicals are rinsed out and the hair retains the shape of being wrapped around the rods. The increased curliness of the hair creates the appearance of greater hair density, and helps to hide the scalp under thinning hair. But perms need to done periodically as the hair grows out and the chemicals used can weaken the hairs and cause increased breakage, and sometimes may cause scalp irritation.

Cutting the hair short is a surprisingly effective solution for moderately thinning hair. Usually the hair on the top of the head gets thinner than the sides and back. When thin hair is allowed to grow long, it can get "stringy", and draws attention to the scalp that is visible under the strands of hair in the thin area. But when all of the hair is worn short, the thin area on top is less apparent. This styling technique can be made even more effective by thinning out the hair on the sides and back adjacent to the thin area on top. Hair stylists have special scissors with comb-shaped blades for thinning hair; or an electric clipper can be used.

And then there is always the option of shaving the head completely. Shaving the head is a bold move, but it solves the hair loss problem completely. Athletes, chemotherapy patients, and people with moderate to severe alopecia areata commonly use this solution. A shaved head also allows for the occasional use of other temporary cosmetic solutions such wigs, hats, and scarves.

Another bold hair styling technique that men can use is to allow facial hair to grow out in order to draw attention away from a receding hairline or bald spot. Moustaches and beards can help to reshape your face, but they're not for everybody. While facial hair can give some men a distinguished look, they can add years to the apparent age of others. And many men simply don't look good with beards or moustaches.

HAIR CARE PRODUCTS

The hair care product industry, like the perfume industry, sells "hope in a bottle." There are countless products claiming to give the look of "fuller, thicker hair." Shampoos and conditioners clean the hair and scalp, remove excess oils, and seal the hair shaft to maintain moisture and keep hair manageable. While some conditioners coat the hair shaft and make the hair more manageable, some people with thin hair find that conditioners flatten their hair making their hair loss even more noticeable. Shampoos without conditioners can result in hair that is "frizzy" and less manageable when worn long. However, when the hair is short this can be a desirable result that gives the appearance of greater hair density.

In addition to shampoos and conditioners, there are thousands of spray-on thickeners, foam mousse products, gels, and lotions that all promise to improve the look of people with thin hair. Many of these products coat the hair shaft, in a manner similar to how mascara thickens eyelashes.

Hair dye and bleaching products can give mixed results. Some feel that for those with light-colored skin, making dark hair lighter can reduce the contrast between the hair and the skin on the scalp, which can make thin hair less apparent. On the other hand, some feel that darkening thin hair can sometimes make what hair exists seem more prominent. In either case, once the hair is colored or bleached, the treatment must be repeated periodically to avoid having different colored roots become visible as the colored hairs grow out.

Scalp coloring cosmetics are types of cosmetic products for treating hair loss that fall into in a category separate from other hair care products. These products color the skin on the scalp, reducing the contrast between the hair and scalp, which otherwise draws attention to thinning hair. Some of these products are heavily pigmented talcum powders in an aerosol spray can, and others are liquid scalp paints, and some are colored lotions that come in squeeze tubes. Scalp coloring products are selected to match the color of the existing hair, and are applied to the skin on the scalp, rather than to the hair itself. These products tend to work best for thinning areas, surrounded by dense hair growth. By covering the scalp with pigment, there is less contrast between the skin and the hair, and what hair exists looks fuller and thicker. Make-up artists use scalp coloring products to prepare actors and actresses for television and film performances. A major disadvantage of scalp cosmetics is that away from the camera, the painted-head look is apparent. Also, some versions of this product are not waterproof, so care must be taken if perspiration is a possibility, or if rain is anticipated. Most scalp paint products can be readily shampooed off in the evening.

Another type of cosmetic treatment for hair loss are dust and fiber products that are sprinkled into the hair, just as artificial snow flocking is sprayed onto Christmas trees. Like scalp paint, the color of the dust or fiber product is selected to match the existing hairs. Dust and fiber products are almost undetectable, even upon close visual inspection, and are ideal for use on camera, even under bright television lighting. Certain dust and fiber products can also be used immediately after hair restoration surgery to effectively camouflage newly-placed hair grafts until they have healed. Regular shampooing rinses the dust and powder away.

HAIRPIECES

Hairpieces are artificial hair devices designed to cover the bald spot on the top or front of the head, and to blend in with a person's existing hair along the sides and back. They can be constructed from natural human hair or synthetic fibers, which are usually placed into a transparent synthetic mesh base. Hairpieces go by many names, including hair appliances, hair extensions, hair weaves, hair systems, units, and non-surgical solutions. Today, hairpieces are usually attached to the scalp by adhesives, or by weaving the person's existing hair through the clear mesh base at the edges of the hairpiece.

Artificial hair will work for just about anyone with hair loss. There is no concern about the degree of effectiveness, which is an issue with medications, or having adequate donor hair, which is a problem with surgical hair restoration.

Hairpieces made from human hair are more costly than synthetic hairpieces, and they require more maintenance. However, when they are constructed carefully and matched well to the individual's existing hair, human hair hairpieces can look very natural. Synthetic hairpieces last longer; however, they generally look and feel less genuine.

Hairpieces have several advantages as a treatment for hair loss. They are relatively fast and easy solutions. There is no waiting for months for medication to work, or for surgically-relocated hair follicles to begin to grow new hair. A custom made hairpiece may take several weeks to complete, but after that you have instant hair.

And hairpieces and wigs can be constructed with whatever hair density is desired. Hairpieces and wigs actually add new hair, while transplant surgery just moves existing hair around. A hair unit that is too thick for the age of the user will look fake, so expertly designed custom hairpieces are made with only moderate hair density. But even these hairpieces are generally constructed with greater hair density than can be achieved with micrograft hair transplants.

Artificial hair will work for just about anyone with hair loss. There is no concern about the degree of effectiveness, which is an issue with medications; or having adequate donor hair, which is a problem with surgical hair restoration.

Hair appliances will work even if you have no hair at all. A hairpiece that covers the entire scalp is called a "wig." Hairpieces and wigs are also ideal for people with temporary hair loss, which may be caused by various diseases, or medical treatments such as chemotherapy or radiation therapy.

But hairpieces also have some distinct disadvantages. By far the most significant disadvantage is fear of detection. While cosmetics for the skin and even tanning bed tans are accepted, there continues to be a certain stigma against wearing artificial hair, regardless of whether it is synthetic or human hair. Wearing a hairpiece is fine, as long as it is not discovered. Despite the perfectly reasonable desire to look one's best, wearing a hairpiece in particular can be embarrassing. It's a "cover-up." It's fake. So artificial hair wearers expend considerable effort to avoid detection.

The first line of defense against detection is the visual appearance of the hairpiece. A hairpiece wearer must be ever vigilant to assure their hairpiece looks natural at all times and well groomed, but not too well groomed. It has to be cleaned and styled to look good...but not too good. The wearer's real growing hair on the back and sides of the head must be trimmed as needed to match the length of the hair in the hairpiece, which obviously does not grow at all.

When the hairpiece wearer begins to develop gray hair, the hairpiece must be altered or replaced to blend in with the changes. And all hairpieces wear out eventually, and must be repaired or replaced periodically before they look too unnatural. Hairpiece users need to have at least two hairpieces, so that they can wear one while the other is being cleaned, modified, or repaired. Most hairpiece users own three or four "units."

The second line of defense against detection is secure attachment, and regular re-attachment. At some point, all hairpiece wearers worry about their hairpiece coming loose. Many methods for attaching hairpieces have been tried in the past, including suturing the unit directly to the scalp, clipping the hairpiece to loops of live skin surgically constructed on the scalp, and even snapping one to bolts screwed through the scalp and anchored into the skull. But the most popular methods today are double-sided tape, weaving, and liquid adhesives. Double-sided tape is fast and clean, and allows a hairpiece to be easily removed at night; however it is the least secure attachment method.

Attachment by weaving is more labor-intensive, but very secure. A hairpiece designed for weaving has very fine clear mesh along the edges, and the person's own hair is pulled through the hairpiece and woven into the mesh to achieve a secure fit. A weave will last for a month or longer, before hair growth begins to loosen the fit of the hairpiece. Weaves require reattachment every four to six weeks, to compensate for the attachment hairs growing out at the rate of about one half inch each month.

Liquid adhesive attachment is also very secure, and allows the hairpiece to remain in place for a month or longer. With adhesive attachment, the scalp is cleaned, adhesive is applied, and the hairpiece is pressed into place. The adhesive is placed in a U-shaped pattern with an opening at the back to allow cleaning the scalp under the hairpiece by using shampoo and a jet of water.

With modern adhesives, the risk of a glued-on hairpiece coming loose prematurely is practically zero. However there is still a limit to how long a hairpiece can remain glued on. Over time the skin cells on the scalp are shed, and glands in the scalp secrete oils, which eventually loosen the adhesive. The dead skin cells and oils can also accumulate under the hairpiece. This can cause bad odors, and in extreme cases, skin irritation.

So a third line of defense against detection is regular hygiene to avoid bad smell and scalp problems. Most hairpiece attachment techniques are designed to allow the wearer to loosen one edge of the hairpiece to wash under it, and then reattach the edge. Those hairpiece users who choose to have their units glued on for a month or longer, must take care to wash under their hairpiece regularly to avoid odors and possible skin irritation and infection.

The final line of defense against detection involves touch. In intimate situations, most hairpiece wearers fear that their hairpiece will feel unnatural to anyone touching their hair, and that discovery during certain situations can be awkward, at best. Many hairpiece wearers avoid letting anyone touch their hair. Hairpieces constructed with human hair generally feel more natural to the touch than synthetics, but most hairpiece wearers agree that discovery by their partner is inevitable, and usually choose to explain their "appliance" at the right moment, before it is discovered.

Surprisingly, cost is another disadvantage of hairpieces. Over time they are the most expensive alternative of all the hair loss treatment methods. While hairpieces are often sold by mail-order and over the Internet for $500-$700, a good quality hairpiece can cost $1,000-$5,000, and usually one or more identical spares are purchased at the same time, so that one can be worn while the other can be cleaned or repaired as necessary.

Hairpieces wear out and need to be replaced every year or two. In addition to the cost of the units, there is also the ongoing cost of service, with periodic visits to the "hair club" for hairpiece removal, scalp and hairpiece cleaning, hair cutting, and hairpiece reattachment. Even for do-it-yourselfers, considerable time is required to maintain a hairpiece in top condition at all times. Over a lifetime, the cost of hairpieces and maintenance is more than the cost of the ongoing medications or the cost of several hair transplant surgery sessions.

Wigs

Wigs cover the entire scalp, and are often preferred by women with overall diffuse hair loss, by people with unpredictable patchy hair loss, and by people with total hair loss. Wigs temporarily replace all the hair on the scalp. Wigs are an excellent cosmetic solution for those with alopecia areata or alopecia totalis, and autoimmune condition that results in partial or full hair loss. Wigs are also prescribed, just like a medication, for chemotherapy patients who are likely to lose their hair as a result of treatment. Wigs can be attached with tape or glue in the same manner as a hairpiece. However, there are also vacuum fit attachment devices designed especially for full-cap wigs that offer the benefit of a very secure and comfortable fit without chemical adhesives.

8

Drugs That Can Cause Hair Loss

PRESCRIPTION DRUGS

There are many categories of prescription drugs that have been reported to cause hair loss, and the medications listed below present a risk of temporary hair loss as a possible side effect. It is important to note that hair loss is only an infrequent possible side effect of these medications, and when it does happen, hair loss may occur after a few weeks or after years of use of a particular drug. Factors such as dosage, duration of treatment, and normal variations in how people respond to medications determine the degree of hair loss that may occur, if any. In most cases, hair growth resumes around three to four months following the discontinuation of the medication.

In addition to the following list of drug types and specific hair loss-causing drug examples, a much longer alphabetical list of drugs that have been reported to cause hair loss appears in Appendix 2.

Certain cholesterol-lowering drugs have hair loss as a possible side effect, including: clofibrate, gemfibrozil (Lopid).

Some Parkinson medications may cause hair loss in some people, including: levodopa (Dopar, Larodopa).

Common ulcer medications that may cause alopecia (hair loss) are: cimetidine (Tagamet), ranitidine (Zantac), and famotidine (Pepcid).

High blood pressure beta-blocker medications that have been noted to occasionally cause hair loss include: Atenolol (Tenormin), metoprolol (Lopressor), nadolol (Corgard), propranolol (Inderal), and timolol (Blocadren)

Common anticoagulants (blood thinners) that cause hair loss are: warfarin, coumarin, and heparin.

A gout medication that may cause hair loss is: allopurinol (Zyloprim).

Arthritis medications that may cause hair loss include: penicillamine, indomethacin (Indocin), naproxen (Naprosyn), sulindac (Clinoril), methotrexate (Folex)

It has already been noted that vitamin A in excessive doses over a period of time can cause hair loss. Some medications that are vitamin A derivatives can also contribute to thinning hair, including: isotretinoin (Accutane), acitretin (Soriatane).

Nonsteroidal anti-inflammatory drugs (NSAIDs) are widely used to treat inflammation, fever, and pain, but in some cases they also cause hair loss. Common over-the-counter NSAIDs such as ibuprofen and naproxen are included in this category of drugs. Prescription NSAIDs that may also cause hair loss include: celecoxib (Celebrex), diclofenac (Voltaren), etodolac (Lodine), fenoprofen (Nalfon), indomethacin (Indocin), ketoprofen (Orudis, Oruvail), oxaprozin (Daypro), nabumetone (Relafen), and sulindac (Clinoril).

Hormone Replacement Therapy drugs, as well as many oral contraceptives (birth control pills), contain progestins, estrogens, and estrogen-like compounds ("female" hormones) that can cause hair loss in some women. It is significant to note that the same medications are frequently prescribed to reverse hair loss, as well. It just happens that in some women, they help stop hair loss, while in others they cause hair thinning.

Anabolic steroids are synthetic androgens commonly referred to as "male hormones." In addition to being prescribed for certain medical conditions, anabolic steroids also have a history of being used by body-builders seeking to increase their muscle mass. In men with a genetic predisposition to hair loss, the excessive use of these medications can cause premature baldness. Testosterone in various forms is used as a medication with brand names including Testex, Depo-Testosterone, and Delatestryl. Other anabolic steroid hormone medications that can cause hair loss include fluoxymesterone (Halotestin), methyltestosterone (Android, Metandren, Oreton, Testred, Virilon), stanozolol (Winstrol), and danazol (Danocrine).

Thyroid gland disorders can result in hair loss; however some thyroid medications such as thiouracil can also cause hair thinning as well.

CHEMOTHERAPY DRUGS

Chemotherapy drug treatment almost always causes hair loss because the drugs target rapidly dividing cells typical of cancer. The cells in a hair follicle that produce the hair shaft also divide rapidly, and actively producing hair follicles are shut down by chemotherapy drugs. This type of hair loss is called anagen effluvium, and it is characterized by relatively sudden and massive hair shedding. Since approximately ninety percent of all hair follicles are actively growing hairs at any given time, with the other ten percent resting or just waiting to shed hairs, the typical effect of chemotherapy drugs is near total hair loss in a short period of time.

When undergoing chemotherapy, hair loss often begins two to three weeks after the first treatment and progresses over the next one to two months. Usually most or all the hair on the scalp is shed, and with prolonged treatment there may also be loss of hair on the face, arms, legs, underarms, and pubic area. The hair usually begins to grow back about three to four months following the last chemotherapy treatment, however hair only grows about one-half inch a month, and it may take several months before good coverage is achieved.

Hair loss from chemotherapy often has a devastating psychological effect on cancer patients, and there have been attempts to reduce the degree of hair loss with various devices and drugs. One method to reduce hair loss involves the application of a tourniquet around the scalp to restrict blood flow during chemotherapy, in an attempt to reduce the amount of chemotherapy drugs received by the hair follicles. Another method involves chilling the scalp with various cooling devices, also to reduce blood flow and limit the effect of the chemotherapy drugs. And there have been advances with medications that temporarily stop the hair follicles from growing hair, and as a result reduce their absorption of the chemotherapy drugs. None of these methods work perfectly, and all can increase the risk of cancer cells surviving in the hair follicles.

Common chemotherapy drugs that routinely cause hair loss include: bleomycin, cyclophosphamide, cytarabine, dactinomycin, daunorubicin, doxorubicin, etoposide, fluorouracil, and methotrexate.

For a complete list, see Appendix 2.

9

Drugs That Grow Hair

Cowntless medications, nutrients, herbs, and chemicals have been claimed to stop or reverse hair loss, however when tested scientifically in well controlled, double blind clinical trials, almost none have been proven to be effective. Of course, hundreds of bogus hair loss products continue to make claims about their effectiveness, including presenting bogus "testimonials" by medical doctors and users, "scientific evidence" of effectiveness, and even fake results from "well controlled, double-blind clinical studies." In the United States alone, hundreds of millions of dollars are wasted each year on "medical" treatments for hair loss products that simply do not work. Bogus hair loss treatments also sell well in Central and South America, in Asia, and Europe.

This chapter reveals the four most effective medications proven scientifically for treating genetic hair loss. All four of these drugs were originally approved by the FDA for treating medical conditions other than hair loss. All can slow the rate of inherited hair loss, and in many cases they can help hair follicles that have recently shut down to begin to grow hair again. Individual results will vary. This chapter also includes a final section on topical treatments.

One medication, Propecia (finasteride), is typically prescribed for men only, due to possible side effects when taken by pregnant women. Another, Rogaine (minoxidil), is useful for treating both men and women. The last two, high-estrogen oral contraceptives and aldactone (spironolactone) are generally prescribed for women only, due to the risk of undesirable feminizing side effects in men.

PROPECIA (FINASTERIDE)

The single most effective medication proven to treat genetic pattern hair loss is Propecia. It is prescribed for men with a genetic predisposition to hair loss (male pattern baldness). Propecia is the brand name for the drug finasteride. Finasteride is a prescription medication that was first approved by the United States Food and Drug Administration (U.S. FDA) for treating enlarged prostate glands. To the delight of some patients taking finasteride for enlarged prostate glands, a side effect of this medication was decreased hair loss, and often re-growth of hair recently lost.

In 1998, after years of additional testing as a hair loss treatment, finasteride was also approved in pill form, at a lower dosage, as an anti-baldness treatment. It is sold as a prescription prostate medication in five-milligram tablet form under the brand name Proscar. For treatment of hair loss, it is sold in one-milligram tablets under the brand name Propecia. For treating baldness, the lower dosage is adequate. The hair loss reduction effect of Propecia occurs at a much lower dosage than that needed to treat enlarged prostrate glands.

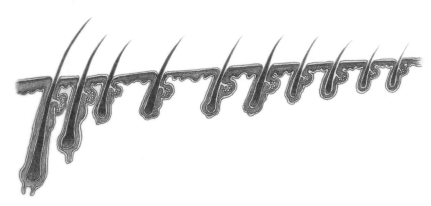

Testosterone ——— **5-alpha-reductase Type II** ——→ **DHT**

Without Propecia, testosterone in the blood is converted freely by the enzyme 5-alpha-reductase into a form of testosterone called dihydrotestosterone (DHT).

Finasteride effectively blocks one form of the 5-alpha-reductase enzyme that converts testosterone into DHT. By blocking the conversion of testosterone into DHT, Propecia prevents the "hair loss message" from getting to hair follicles that are genetically programmed to be sensitive to DHT. This helps stop further hair loss, and in many cases regular Propecia use actually results in significant hair re-growth of recently lost hairs.

Without Propecia, testosterone in the blood is converted freely by the enzyme 5-alpha-reductase into a form of testosterone called dihydrotestosterone (DHT). In men susceptible to pattern hair loss, certain scalp hair follicles are genetically predisposed to respond in a negative ways to elevated levels of DHT in the bloodstream. The most susceptible hair follicles are typically located at the temples, front, and top of the head, but all hair follicles may eventually be influenced to some degree by normal DHT levels. One negative response to DHT is a shortening of the growing phase of the hair follicles, and another is the progressive miniaturization of the hair follicles, which causes miniaturization of the hairs they produce. The end result is shorter and smaller hairs, and fewer and fewer hair follicles producing hairs.

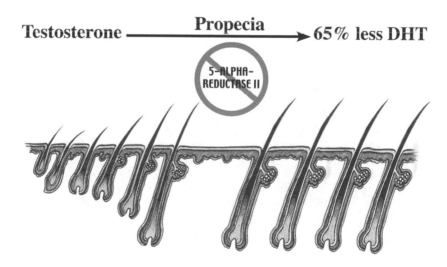

Propecia blocks a form of 5-alpha-reductase found primarily in the prostate gland, called type-II 5-alpha-reductase, from converting testosterone to DHT.

Propecia blocks a form of 5-alpha-reductase found primarily in the prostate gland, called type-II 5-alpha-reductase, from converting testosterone to DHT. The result is lower levels of DHT in the blood. Over many years, DHT in the bloodstream signals hair follicles to shorten their growing phase and to miniaturize. By reducing the amount of DHT in the blood, Propecia reduces the strength of the DHT hormone message, so many of the follicles that would have quit instead continue to produce new hairs.

Continuous treatment is required to maintain this benefit, as 5-alpha-reductase will continue converting testosterone to DHT if treatment is discontinued. However the benefit of using Propecia for any period of time is still realized; Propecia buys time for men with a genetic predisposition for hair loss. The DHT message to stop growing hair must continue for many years, and often many decades, for DHT-sensitive hair follicles to get the message and stop growing new hairs. If the DHT message is disrupted for a period of time, the clock is stopped. In other words, if a thirty-year-old man who would lose his hair by age sixty uses Propecia for twenty years and then stops, he will delay the age when he would lose his hair to age eighty. The benefit of using Propecia for twenty years is not lost when use is discontinued.

With Propecia use, the rate of hair loss slows, and in many cases stops. In many individuals, some recently miniaturized hair follicles begin to grow back to normal size, and begin to grow normal size hairs again. This results in increased hair. The degree of hair regrowth can vary from no measurable regrowth, to significant regrowth.

Double blind clinical tests have shown that Propecia helps men keep the hair they have. In one two-year study, eighty-three percent of men taking Propecia maintained their hair at the top of their heads (vertex area), compared to twenty-eight percent of men taking a placebo. In the same study, seventeen percent of the men taking Propecia still experienced measurable hair loss, but seventy two percent of the men taking the placebo also experienced additional hair loss. After the first two years, results of the group taking Propecia continued to improve.

In addition to stopping further hair loss, Propecia can also help regrow recently lost hair. In another two-year clinical trial, sixty-six percent of men taking Propecia had measurable hair regrowth at the vertex, while only seven percent of men taking a placebo had regrowth. In this study, only one percent of men taking Propecia continued to have hair loss at the top of their heads, while thirty-three percent of men taking a placebo showed a decreased hair count in this area.

For many years before it was approved as a hair loss treatment, a level of safety has been established for finasteride, the active ingredient in Propecia. As a prescription drug already approved by the FDA for treating enlarged prostate glands, it has been extensively researched and tested. Based on studies of hormone breakdown products found in the urine, it seems to affect only the 5-alpha-reductase enzyme, and not other hormones in the blood such as testosterone. Propecia is not an antiandrogen. In fact, levels of testosterone in the blood often increase by ten to fifteen percent when taking Propecia.

Finasteride has been shown to be effective at stopping hair loss when taken by mouth in tablet form at much smaller doses than that used to treat enlarged prostate glands. Some possible side effects of finasteride treatment for hair loss may be seen as beneficial, such as possible shrinking of the prostate gland in men susceptible to an enlarged prostate. My personal theory is that taking the lower dosage of finasteride in Propecia early in life may protect men with a genetic predisposition from suffering enlarged prostate glands and prostate cancer as they get older.

A single one milligram Propecia tablet taken daily is the usual prescribed dose for hair loss treatment. Propecia is a treatment, not a cure. This means that a pill must be taken every day for the benefits to continue. When Propecia is discontinued, the hair loss process resumes.

Propecia is for men only, and is not approved by the FDA as a hair loss treatment for women or children. A woman taking finasteride would have only a small decrease DHT levels because most of the effect of finasteride is on type-II 5-alpha-reductase that is primarily made in prostate glands. Women who take finasteride and become pregnant may cause a male fetus to develop ambiguous genitals, and have female characteristics until puberty (at puberty, the child's genitals normalize).

Propecia treatment may cause a loss of sex drive in one to two percent of patients as a result of reducing levels of DHT circulating in the blood. Treatment with Viagra can be helpful in these cases. Discontinuing Propecia eliminates this possible side effect, if it occurs.

There is also a small risk of reducing the volume of ejaculate if the prostate gland is reduced in size as a result of Propecia treatment. Sperm activity remains normal. Discontinuing Propecia eliminates this possible side effect.

Both of these conditions can affect up to two percent of men in the first month of use, but drop to about a half percent when measured again after two years.

The story of finasteride begins with scientists who were working with a family in the Dominican Republic who had a genetic trait that caused them to give birth to male children with ambiguous genitalia. Female babies were not affected. In many cases it was difficult to determine such an infant's gender by observation alone. At puberty, when hormone levels in these affected individuals increased, these young boys normalized. They eventually had children of their own, and perpetuated the genetic trait.

It was observed that the adult males in this group being studied did not suffer from enlarged prostate glands, never developed prostate cancer, nor did they lose their hair. No male pattern baldness! Genetic research showed that their gene for producing the 5-alpha-reductase enzyme was inactive. With no 5-alpha-reductase enzyme, testosterone in the blood was not readily converted to DHT. The low levels of DHT that resulted prevented their hair follicles from getting the message to have shorter growth cycles and miniaturization.

Scientists figured that if they could create a medication to regulate the activity of 5-alpha-reductase they could accomplish some of the positive effects of this genetic trait, such as prostate gland normalization and, later hair loss prevention.

Merck, the maker of Proscar for the prostate and Propecia for hair loss, has taken the stance that women shouldn't touch the pill or the bottle if they are pregnant, and they should not have sex with men who are taking the medication. The rationale behind this is that

5-alpha-reductase, if inhibited in a developing fetus, might result in a male child with a very small penis. People who are missing the enzyme 5-alpha-reductase type II—and there are families of them—have boys who are born looking like little girls. But at age twelve, the testicles descend and they become men. Given the facts, Merck put a warning on their bottles of Proscar and Propecia. Although this defies logic and may sound ludicrous (even if it was radioactive you'd have a hard time measuring it and a woman would have to have gallons and gallons of semen to absorb enough to measure it), Merck did not want to take the risk. Compare this to the warning on a bottle of Jim Beam. It does not say women should not have sex with drunk men, it says pregnant women should not get drunk. However, no doctor—including me—would tell a male patient it is perfectly safe to use Proscar or Propecia and then have sex with a pregnant wife because a certain number of boys are born with this birth abnormality for unknown reasons and it could be blamed on the drug.

Avodart, dutasteride, was released at the end of 2001 for treatment of benign prostate hypertrophy. It blocks both Type I and II 5-alpha-reductase and lowers DHT by over ninety-five percent in men, whereas Propecia lowers it only sixty-six percent. Type II is found in the prostate gland and Type I in skin and hair. Women only have type II, therefore women with thinning hair may benefit from Dutasteride. I routinely place my male patients on Dutasteride if they are part of the small group who continue to lose hair while on Propecia.

Dutasteride is currently being studied for hair loss, but results have not yet been published.

ROGAINE (MINOXIDIL)

After years of testing and clinical trials, in 1988, Rogaine topical lotion became the first medication approved by the FDA for treating genetic hair loss. The medication is a colorless and odorless liquid applied to the scalp. Rogaine is the brand name for the drug minoxidil when used as a hair loss treatment in lotion form. Before 1988, minoxidil had already been FDA approved in pill form as a prescription medication for treating high blood pressure. The brand name for minoxidil pills is Loniten.

Research on minoxidil's potential as an anti-baldness medication started after some Loniten patients noticed substantial new hair growth, a condition doctors call hypertrichosis. Usually the new hair growth was on the head and was desirable, but in some cases it also occurred on the arms, back, chest, and other areas. So researchers worked on a lotion form of the medication that could be applied to the scalp or face to direct new hair growth only where it was wanted.

Starting in 1988, Rogaine lotion was available only by prescription, and only in a two percent concentration. In 1995, the FDA decided minoxidil lotion was adequately safe for use without a prescription and Rogaine was soon available over-the-counter in pharmacies and grocery stores. Generic versions of Rogaine became available when the patent on minoxidil expired, and the range of concentrations increased up to five percent. Most people using minoxidil lotion choose the five percent strength lotion, because it produces slightly faster results than the two percent concentration.

Researchers are not certain exactly how minoxidil works to stop hair loss or increase hair growth. It is known that it does not affect DHT levels in the blood. Minoxidil is a vasodilator, meaning it helps blood vessels enlarge. Other vasodilators, however, do not stop hair loss or increase hair growth.

Minoxidil lotion seems to work only on active hair follicles still capable of producing some hair, even if the hair produced is just "peach fuzz." One symptom of people with genetic pattern hair loss is the progressive miniaturization of hair follicles at the end of each growth cycle, resulting in finer and finer hairs being produced.

Minoxidil seems to reduce the rate of hair follicle miniaturization, and can cause hair follicles that formerly produced full-size hairs, but have recently become miniaturized, to increase in size and begin to grow full size hairs again. Also, the enlarged follicles seem to remain in the anagen, or growth stage for a longer period. A longer growth period results in the production of longer hairs, and a look of more hair. Minoxidil acts as "life support" for hair follicles.

Results with minoxidil vary. For some people, it seems to have no effect at all. For others there is reduced rate of hair loss, but no visible new hair growth. Some men and women experience minimal new hair growth, but not enough to cover thin hair areas. Others enjoy dense new hair growth with areas that had previously been thin developing hair density similar to areas that were not affected by hair loss.

Clinical studies were run during which some men and women with pattern hair loss applied Rogaine to their scalps, and others with pattern hair loss applied a placebo: the same mixture of water, alcohol, and propylene glycol used in Rogaine, but without the minoxidil. The men and women selected for the study had thin hair or baldness on the top of their heads, where minoxidil is most effective at promoting hair regrowth. The effectiveness of the minoxidil treatment was compared to the placebo lotion. The results of clinical studies involving thousands of men and women have shown Rogaine is able to produce a statistically significant increase in hair regrowth.

Those likely to achieve the best results with Rogaine are in the early stages of pattern hair loss. On the average, younger people get better results than older people. Those with thinning or baldness on the top of their heads generally get better results than those with hair loss at the hairline. People with diffuse hair loss, especially women, tend to get better results than those with clear bald spots. Those with smaller bald spots usually show more regrowth than those with large bald spots.

Minoxidil lotion is applied on the scalp two times each day. The lotion form of the drug causes the hair-growing effect to take place on the scalp only, and not on other parts of the body. There is no effect on blood pressure when applied as directed. Rogaine is a treatment, not a cure. This means that the lotion must be applied to the scalp twice a day for the benefits to continue. Skipping a day or two occasionally is not likely to cause any measurable difference in the effectiveness of minoxidil treatment. After several months of discontinued use, however the regrown hairs are likely to be shed.

Also, for those who discontinue the minoxidil for a few months the hairs that would have been shed if the minoxidil had not prevented follicle miniaturization will also be lost as those follicles begin to shrink. So both regrown hairs and hairs that would have otherwise been lost if not for the minoxidil use may be shed within just a few months after discontinuing use.

Minoxidil lotion is safe. When used as directed and applied to the scalp, only very small amounts of it reach the blood. The risk of serious side effects is very small.

Hair transplant patients can use minoxidil. Many surgeons recommend using it within a few weeks after surgery to promote the growth of the transplanted hair follicles. Minoxidil may also help reduce the tendency for mini and micro grafts to temporarily enter the telogen, or rest phase, immediately after being transplanted.

The most common side effect when used as directed is minor scalp irritation. In clinical studies involving 6,000 men and women about seven percent of those using two percent strength Rogaine lotion experienced some degree of scalp itching, inflammation, dryness, or flaking. A smaller percentage of patients experience an increased pulse rate.

Some women using extra strength minoxidil lotion (five percent) experience increased facial hair growth. This side effect tends to diminish after the first few months of treatment, or two percent minoxidil can be used. When treatment is discontinued normal facial hair growth resumes.

Minoxidil treatment does not work on everybody with thinning hair due to inherited pattern hair loss. It is less effective for hair loss at the hairline than on the top of the head. It is less effective on large bald spots than small ones. It is less effective on small bald spots than on diffuse thin areas. It is less effective on long-established shiny bald areas than those with recent hair loss.

Minoxidil takes time to produce results. When two percent minoxidil is used twice daily, a gradual change in appearance occurs in a matter of months; five percent minoxidil produces slightly faster results. Several months are usually required before significant benefit can be seen. The results may improve further over the next several months with continuous twice-daily use. The maximum benefit is usually achieved after about twelve months of minoxidil use, and at that point hair regrowth tends to stabilize.

Some dermatologists prepare custom-blended minoxidil lotion, with added ingredients to reduce the risk of inflammation and increase absorption. One such additive is tretinoin (Retin-A): Tretinoin is a prescription acne medication applied to the skin, and is also well known for helping to reduce facial wrinkles. Minoxidil lotion applied with low concentrations of tretinoin has been show to promote greater hair growth—and possibly faster results—than minoxidil used alone. Tretinoin may increase the absorption of minoxidil through the skin as well as having additional hair growth promoting effects. In addition to the risks and advantages of minoxidil use, however tretinoin adds additional risk of skin irritation and inflammation.

Another minoxidil lotion additive is betamethasone valerate, a cortisone medication that helps to prevent scalp inflammation. In addition to reducing possible scalp irritation, it may also enhance the hair restoration effect of minoxidil in two ways: first, it helps block the metabolism of testosterone in the cells of the hair follicle where the hormone signal to "stop producing new hairs" takes place. Blocking this signal may keep more hairs growing. Second, betamethasone valerate helps to disperse the white blood cells that are called up to push the hair shaft out. In doing so, the white blood cells scar the hair follicle, reducing to a degree the follicle's ability to produce new hairs. By reducing scarring, betamethasone valerate may help keep the hair follicles active for more hair growth cycles. Male pattern baldness is a scarring alopecia, and the betamethasone valerate helps reduce scarring of the hair follicle.

Minoxidil lotion can be used at the same time as Propecia pills. The results are better than when either medication used alone.

HIGH ESTROGEN ORAL CONTRACEPTIVES

Women inherit a tendency for pattern hair loss just as men do. But in women the DHT message is usually blocked by relatively high levels of estrogens circulating in the blood. Estrogen levels begin to decline as women begin perimenopause around age forty, and by age fifty-five to fifty-eight most women are in menopause. While testosterone levels usually decline along with progesterone and estrogen, the DHT message may finally start to get through, and thinning hair can result.

Birth control pills contain a combination of synthetic estrogen and progesterone hormones. Since they were first introduced in 1960, the estrogen component of oral contraceptives has been reduced from

.150 milligrams per pill to .020-.035 milligrams. A birth control pill with .035 milligrams of estrogen is considered a "high-estrogen" oral contraceptive. And for reference, the estrogen level in oral contraceptives is several times higher than that of most estrogen replacement medications prescribed for certain women after menopause.

Higher estrogen oral contraceptives such as Ortho Tri-Cyclen or Ortho Novum often work well to inhibit production of androgens (including testosterone) by the ovaries and adrenal glands, which results in lower levels of DHT, therefor, and these stops hair thinning.

Management of women's hormone levels is neither an easy task, nor one where medications are prescribed without careful consideration of the range of benefits and risks.

In addition to reducing androgenetic hair loss, the benefits of taking birth control pills include reduction of the risk of pregnancy, improved skin tone, reduced acne, and for women beginning the first stages of menopause, increased bone mass, decreased occurrence of hot flashes, somewhat tempered mood swings, and reduced irritability.

The risks of taking oral contraceptives include elevated risk of endometrial (uterine) cancer, and, for older women, an increased risk of cardiovascular complications such as heart attacks and strokes. There may also be a slightly elevated risk of breast cancer.

ALDACTONE (SPIRONOLACTONE)

Aldactone is the brand name for spironolactone, a prescription medication used in pill form for treating women with three common problems seen by dermatologists: acne, hirsutism (too much hair, especially on the face), and androgenetic alopecia. The March 2005 *British Journal of Dermatology* reported on a study that showed eighty percent of women receiving oral antiandrogens (spironolcatone) could expect to see no progression of their female pattern hair loss, improved chance of stopping their hair loss, or getting some hair back, after taking the medication for a year at 200 milligrams per day.

Spironolactone is for women what Propecia is for men in preventing hair loss with about the same success rate. A potent anti-androgen, spironolactone binds to DHT receptor sites on hair follicles, thereby blocking DHT from getting its hair loss message to the follicles. This medication is used only for women with androgenetic alopecia (genetic pattern hair loss), because it can produce undesirable side effects in men.

When used as a hair loss treatment, spironolactone is taken as a pill or made into a lotion that is applied directly to the scalp, usually along with minoxidil.

One disadvantage to spironolactone lotion is a disagreeable smell, which is made worse when combined in the same container with Rogaine.

Topical Treatments

A study conducted three years ago using a one percent Zinc Pyrithione ZnP solution daily to the scalp showed that subjects had thicker hair twelve months later. ZnP is the active ingredient in Head and Shoulders shampoo and I advise all my patients with hair loss to use a shampoo with ZnP. Neutrogena makes one called T-Gel Daily with ZnP. The study concluded that Zinc Pyrithione kills bacteria and yeast in the oil glands and hair follicles leading to healthier hairs. Another possibility is that the Zinc itself may inhibit 5-alpha-reductase in the hair follicle.

Last year there was a report of one percent melatonin applied to the scalp of post menopausal women, resulting in thicker hair after twelve months of use. There is no known mechanism for why it works.

Other topical medications that could be incorporated into a topical lotion to block the androgen receptor site are spironolactone, progesterone, zinc salts, azelaic acid, flutamide, dutasteride, and finasteride. Still another study applying a betamethasone valerate (cortisone) solution daily for a year led to thicker hair. Many doctors who specialize in hair loss make up their own prescription blend of a few or most of medications listed above. These medications are often added to a minoxidil solution, and the whole blend can be applied once or twice a day.

10

Surgical Hair Restoration Principles

S urgical forms of hair restoration have had a long history of popularity, mainly because the results are permanent. Once the surgery has been completed and everything has healed, there is no worrying about having a hairpiece discovered, or applying lotions, or taking pills.

But there is a lot of confusion and misinformation about hair restoration surgery. This chapter presents three foundation principles for all hair restoration surgery. Chapter 11 will briefly review the history of hair restoration surgery, with an emphasis on how the techniques used have evolved and improved over time. In Chapter 12, "Follicular Unit Micrografting," I will describe the current state-of-the-art surgical hair restoration technique.

All surgical hair restoration techniques, from old-style "plugs" to state-of-the-art follicular unit micrografting, involve the same medical and artistic principles. The different techniques employ these principles with the goal of achieving the same result: a natural-appearing fuller head of hair.

Any person considering hair restoration surgery will benefit from an understanding of these medical and artistic principles. As a result, they will better understand the benefits and limitations of whatever surgical hair restoration technique they select.

The first principle of hair restoration surgery is called autografting, and it identifies the source of the hair follicles used to correct hair loss—the source is always the patient getting the surgery. The person receiving the surgery is always his or her own "donor," meaning that instead of receiving hair follicles from someone else, they are always taken from a "donor" area on the same person having the surgical procedure.

Nobody has to die in an automobile accident in order to supply the new hair for hair restoration surgery. Self-donation of tissue for surgery eliminates the vast majority of complications that transplantation procedures using tissue donated from others may have, such as costly tissue-matching tests, organ and tissue banks, rejection of the donor tissue, and the need for immune system suppression drugs. These complications simply don't occur with hair transplants or other forms of hair restoration surgery.

The second principal is called donor dominance. This means that the genetic programming for hair growth in the hair follicles that are donated is "dominant" over the conditions where the follicles are moved to. The new donor hair follicles will keep growing new hairs even if relocated to an area where all the existing hair follicles have already shut down.

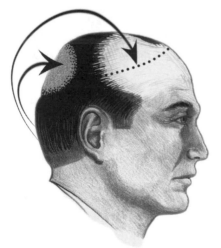 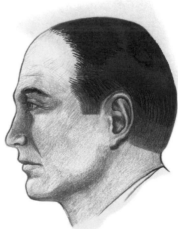

Autografting: the patient is his own donor.

One year afer 1600 grafts

The hair follicles that are selected for donation are the ones that are genetically programmed to continue growing hairs over a lifetime, because they are genetically programmed to be resistant to the DHT message to stop growing hairs. While there currently is no test for hair follicles to determine the degree of susceptibility to DHT, there is a pattern that indicates where the susceptible hair follicles and the resistant hair follicles are usually located (hence the phrase "pattern baldness."). The donor area is the place where baldness does not occur!

Typically, the donor area is at the lower part of the back of the scalp, and extends around to the low part along the sides of the scalp. A key aspect of donor dominance is that only the hair follicles located in the donor area are useful as donor follicles, because they are the ones that are DHT-resistant, and because there is a limited supply of them.

The third principal for all surgical hair restoration surgery is an artistic one, and it follows from the first two principles: self-donation of hair follicles, and choosing only those follicles for donation that are genetically programmed for DHT-resistance. No new hair is added

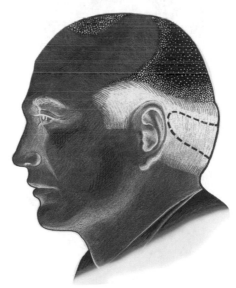

Donor dominance: the white area shows where the DHT-resistant follicles are. The dashed line shows the typical donor area for harvesting follicles for hair transplantation.

with any type of hair restoration surgery, and, of the hair that is available on a patient, only a fraction of that is genetically programmed for DHT-resistance. There is always a very limited supply of donor hair follicles. So the third principal of hair restoration surgery is artistic, and it requires the hair restoration surgeon to redistribute the patient's limited supply of hair follicles on the scalp to give the illusion that there is a fuller head of hair. The hair follicles are relocated, but no new hair is added. The art of hair restoration surgery is creating the illusion of a full head of hair with a limited supply of donor hair follicles.

This artistic principle is even more complicated than it may initially appear, because the surgeon must look decades ahead into the future to plan for future hair loss. On a younger person with only a slightly receding hairline or a small bald spot, it may seem like there

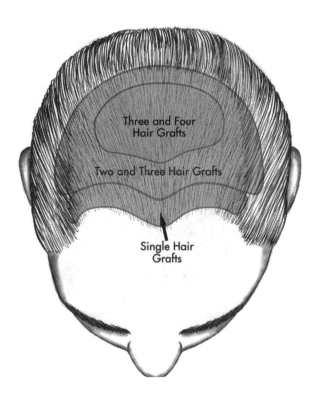

Artistry: placement of hair follicles to achieve the greatest visual impact.
Single hair grafts in front and two to three hair grafts behind.

is a lot of hair to work with to fix the problem. But an experienced hair restoration surgeon knows there is always a very limited supply of donor hair to work with.

Pattern baldness is a progressive condition, meaning that hair loss will continue as the person ages. It may continue at a slow rate, or baldness may progress rapidly. Either way, without the use of medication to slow hair loss, hair loss will increase with age. And people are now living longer than ever. If the patient lives long enough, it is possible that only a fringe of "permanent" hair will continue to grow on the lower sides and back of the head. So it is critical that the precious donor follicles taken from these areas of "permanent hairs" are used effectively. In addition to basic surgical competence, this takes artistry.

The artistic aspect of hair restoration surgery is not often discussed, but it is one of the most important considerations for achieving natural-looking results, especially decades after the procedures are performed. A skilled hair restoration surgeon will certainly avoid medical complications such as infections, excessive scars, and loss of donor hair follicles. But a skilled artistic surgeon will do all that and make the newly relocated hair follicles look as if they are part of a full head of naturally growing hairs. Furthermore, the transplanted hair will continue to look natural decades later, based on an assessment of the patient's future pattern of likely hair loss.

"It is not the paint, nor the brush that makes a great painting...it is the artist."

These three principles: self-donation of hair follicles, donor-dominance of the limited supply of follicles on the sides and back of the head, and the artistic placement of the donor follicles to create a look of having more hair, form the foundation for all hair restoration surgical methods, both past and present.

The following pages show before and after shots of patients undergoing hair transplant surgery.

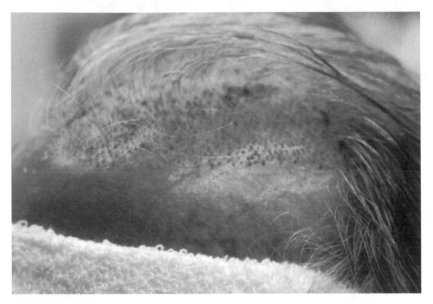

Immediately after grafting—a seventy-one year old man

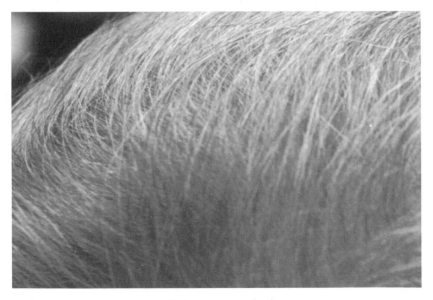

Eighteen months later

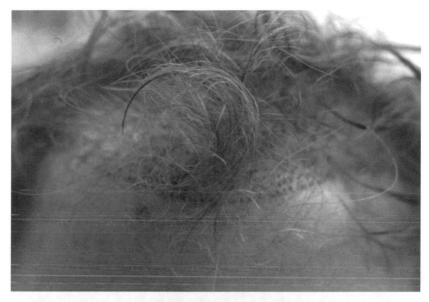

Immediately after 1400 grafts

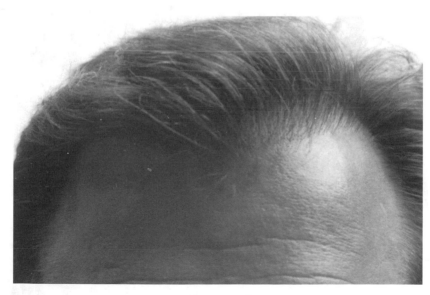

One year later

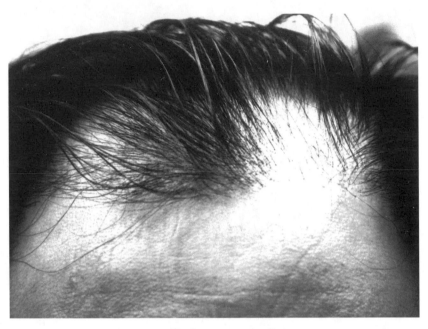

Before 1400 grafts

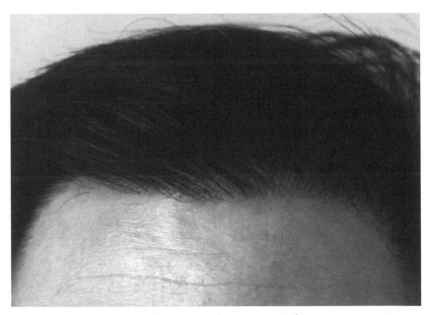

One year after 2000 grafts

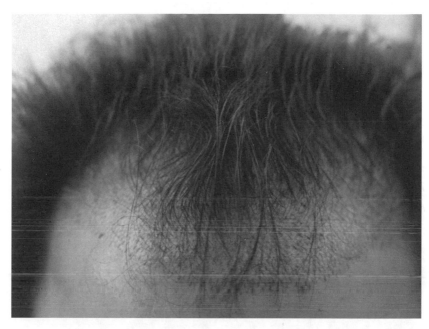

Immediately after 1200 grafts

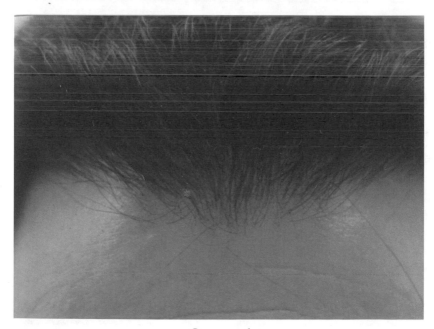

One year later

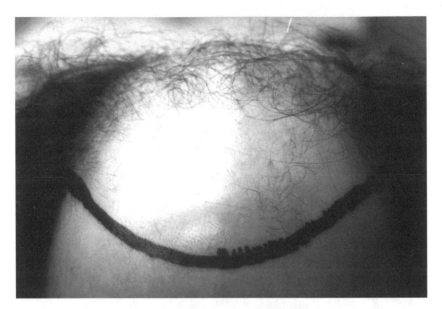

Line marking future of hairline

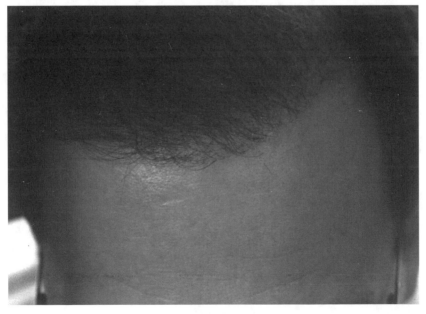

One year after 2000 grafts

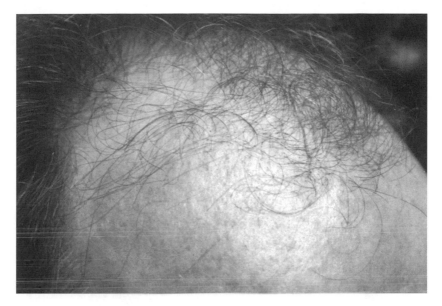

Before 1400 grafts

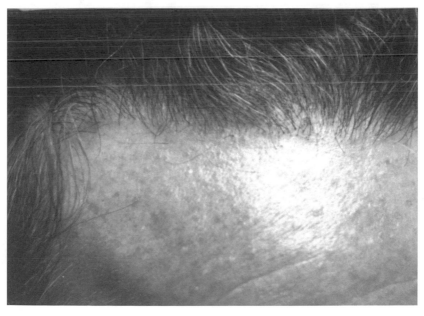

One year later

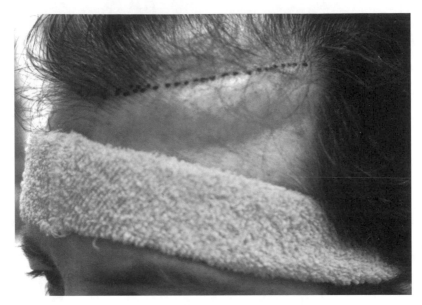

Immediately after 1500 grafts

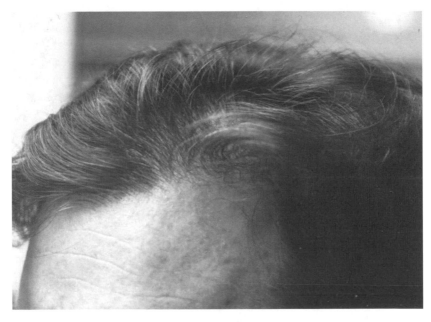

Two years later

11

History of Surgical Hair Restoration

T his chapter reviews the history of some older-style hair restoration surgical methods, including full-size punch grafts, scalp reductions, and scalp lift and flap surgery. Each of these types of older-style surgical methods attempted to address the problem of hair loss by slightly different applications of the three foundation principles of surgical hair restoration: autografting, donor dominance, and surgical artistry.

Over the years, as these surgical techniques became more refined and technology advanced, the results from these methods improved. Today, however, they are infrequently performed, and have all been pretty much replaced by the surgical technique called micrografting. They have been replaced by the latest state-of-the-art variation called follicular unit micrografting, which is presented in the next chapter.

When the words "hair transplant" are mentioned, many people still visualize the "pluggy" dolls-hair effect resulting from a single procedure of punch graft hair transplants. Punch grafts, or what are called full-size grafts by hair restoration surgeons, are commonly referred to as "plugs" by people who aren't in the hair restoration surgery business. This type of hair restoration technique was the leading method for many years, but has rarely been performed since the 1980s.

"Plugs" have actually had a very good history of success, despite the technique continuing to be a source of bad jokes and stories. Over a forty-year period, hundreds of thousands of men have enjoyed the benefits of finishing a complete series of full-size hair transplant

Full Size Punch Grafts ("Plugs")

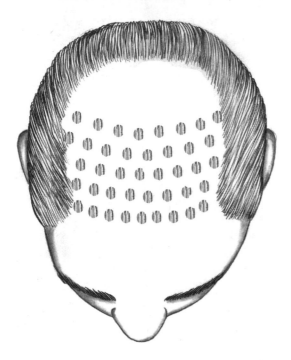

After a single session of full size punch grafts.

sessions performed by skilled and artistic surgeons. Their results are nearly undetectable, and that is the whole idea. Most of the jokes and stories apply to patients who had not completed the full series of procedures, or who have had the misfortune to select less skilled or less artistic surgeons. The full-size graft patients who completed the entire series of procedures, and who had skilled and artistic surgeons, simply look like they have a full head of hair.

The history of this method of surgery began with Dr. Shoji Okuda, a dermatologist in Japan who successfully performed hair transplantation surgery in the 1930s. In 1939, a Japanese medical journal published a description of his technique of using small circular punches to remove donor skin containing hair follicles from the back and sides of the scalp of his patients. Dr. Okuda used the small circular hair-bearing grafts to artistically restore hair on his patient's scalps, eyebrows, and pubic hair regions. Due to World War II, his work was largely unnoticed by dermatologists outside of Japan. A decade passed with minimal public awareness of hair transplantation.

Then, in the 1950s, noted New York dermatologist Dr. Norman Orentreich experimented with hair restoration using punch grafts and reported his findings in American medical journals. He was unaware of Dr. Okuda's earlier work. There was great interest in the procedure. From the late 1950s to the late 1980s, Orentreich's method of punch grafting was the standard method for hair transplantation.

A full-size graft hair transplant procedure was performed under local anesthetic, meaning the scalp was numbed and the patient was awake during surgery. Fifty to one hundred small circular grafts, each about the size of a split pea and containing seven to fifteen hairs each were removed from the back of the head with a circular punch called a trephine. An equal number of small holes were made at the recipient site, starting with the front

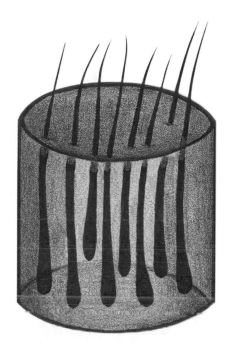

A full size graft.

of the scalp to establish the hairline. Each hole was carefully spaced apart from its neighbors to best assure adequate nutrition for the grafts. The grafts were then placed into the recipient site holes and allowed to heal. The entire procedure took two to three hours. After a three-month wait, another procedure was performed, and another 50-100 grafts were harvested and placed. The spacing between grafts caused the "dolls hair" look after the first procedure. Subsequent procedures filled in the spaces. After four to five procedures the spaces between the recipient sites were completely filled in with growing hair. After the entire series of four to five full size graft hair transplants procedures were done and the last set of grafts had healed, the results were excellent. The patient had a full head of dense growing hair with a solid looking hairline. By the late 1970s, full size graft hair transplants procedures were the most frequently performed elective cosmetic surgical procedure on men. The procedure also enjoyed the highest patient satisfaction rating of any elective cosmetic surgical procedure.

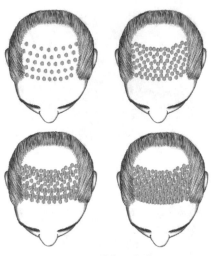

A series of four full-size graft procedures.

But there were also some significant problems with full size graft hair transplants procedures. Perhaps the most significant was the "under construction look" that followed after surgery. Immediately after surgery the grafts were quite evident and bandages, crusts from dried blood, and visible sutures would affect the patients appearance for a couple of weeks. A few patients had adequate hair to comb over the new grafts, others wore a hat or hairpiece temporarily, and some just stayed home and took several days off work until the bandages could be removed.

But even after the grafts had healed and new hairs were growing in, the full size grafts still resulted in an "under construction" look. After the first couple of procedures, the spacing between the grafts created a somewhat unnatural look, like doll's hair, or rows of corn. There was often an uncomfortable six months from the first procedure until after the second procedure healed and the hairs grew enough to effectively cover the spaces between grafts. Subsequent procedures eventually filled in these spaces, but until they were done and the hairs grew long enough, there was an unnatural look. It was this temporary "unfinished" look that caused people to believe they could spot hair transplants because they looked "pluggy." Once all the procedures were accomplished, however, it was nearly impossible to know.

Another disadvantage of full size grafts was that they could only be used for a relatively small bald spot, because the way the individual grafts were harvested severely limited the amount of donor material available, and the grafts had to be placed close together, with several procedures, to achieve a dense natural look.

Problems occurred when full size grafts were used in an attempt to cover too large an area. At some point the donor area at the back of the head could no longer provide additional grafts. The result was either noticeable spaces between the grafts, or the risk of a Swiss cheese look on the back of the head.

There was also the risk of poor results. Inexperienced surgeons could easily misjudge the future extent of baldness when planning a full size graft program. For example, four procedures of 100 grafts may have been the limit of what the donor area could supply, and would have been just enough to cover a thirty-five-year-old man's bald spot. But when the same patient reached age fifty, his hair loss would have progressed further, and the dense full size grafts would become a hairy island on the top of his head, surrounded by recent baldness.

With any surgical procedure there were medical and surgical risks. Serious complications were rare in full-size graft procedures, however, certain problems did arise on occasion. If the hair follicles in the grafts were injured during removal, or while being prepared for insertion, or if too many grafts were placed at one time, some follicles did not survive. These grafts were replaced by new grafts in subsequent procedures. Loss of donor hair was unusual for experienced surgeons.

There was also the risk of visible scars. Anytime the skin is cut, there is risk of a scar. There was the risk of visible scarring with full size grafting at both the donor sites and the recipient sites. Small scars were left at each donor site, where a single small graft was removed. If too many donor "plugs" were removed from donor area at the back of the head, or if the pattern of hair loss continued to advance to an extreme degree, the hair on the back of the head became thinner and as a result did not cover the donor scars as well. As a result, visible scars on the back of the head could create a "Swiss cheese" look.

There was also the risk of scars being visible at the recipient sites, where the grafts were placed, although this was not usually a problem because the hair growing from the new grafts covered any visible scars, and there was always enough donor hair left to cover a few failed graft sites. Another problem with visible scars could result from improperly placed grafts that had to be removed. Some surgeons lacking artistic judgment placed full size grafts too low on the forehead, or they filled in the temples, creating an unnatural look. Removal of these misplaced grafts resulted in fine hairline scars.

Pain was a minor disadvantage with full size graft procedures, and patients were provided with pain-relieving pills. There was some soreness for a couple of weeks at the donor area, when pressure was applied. Most patients went back to work the following day.

Full size graft procedures were costly, with prices ranging from twenty-five to fifty dollars per graft and a total of 300-500 grafts placed over several procedures. This would total between $7,500-25,000 for the full set of procedures. And those were 1980 dollars.

Refinements in full size graft procedures occurred over time, including using sutures to close the donor area wounds, cutting grafts into sections to make mini-grafts for a softer and more natural appearing hairline, and performing a series of scalp reduction procedures before placing grafts into the recipient area.

Scalp reductions lifted the permanent hair growing fringe up toward the top, reducing the size of the bald spot, both at the time of surgery and for the future. When full-size grafts were the only technique, scalp reductions were often the difference between an individual not being a candidate for transplants, and becoming a candidate.

SCALP REDUCTIONS

Scalp reductions had been performed since the 1920s for tumor and scar removal, and from the 1960s through the 1970s, as a way to reduce the amount of bald area needing full-size hair transplant grafts.

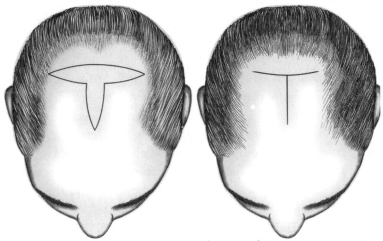

Scalp reduction: before and after.

A scalp reduction allowed the surgeon to place more of the limited supply of donor follicles at the hairline, rather than spreading them over a larger bald area on top. Reductions were also used on occasion in the 1970s to remove chronically inflamed portions of the scalp on people who had tried synthetic fiber artificial hair implants.

While no longer commonly performed for baldness reduction, the procedure is still occasionally done to removed tissue damaged by injury, for skin tumor removal, or for certain cosmetic reasons. Reduction procedures have also been used to repair the appearance of people who have suffered traumatic injury to their scalp from automobile accidents or burns.

Scalp reductions were regularly performed on patients with extensive baldness to improve their condition for hair transplantation. They are rarely performed today. A scalp reduction is the surgical removal of a portion of the bald part of the scalp, performed under local anesthetic. After the portion of bald scalp is removed, the edges of the opening are drawn together so that the adjacent hair-bearing scalp is stretched up or over toward the center of the reduction area. The hair-bearing scalp surrounding the reduction site is stretched slightly as the scalp reduction opening is closed, essentially spread-

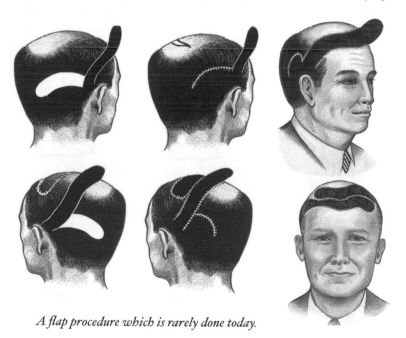

A flap procedure which is rarely done today.

ing the active hair follicles over a larger area. The scalp usually has plenty of flexibility and stretch to allow a strip or T-shaped piece of bald skin an inch or so wide, and five inches long, to be removed in one procedure.

To prepare the scalp for hair restoration surgery, more than one scalp reduction procedure could be performed. Scalp reductions could be repeated every three to four months, further reducing the size of the bald spot each time. With each successive procedure, the fine scar remaining from the previous procedure would be removed along with additional bald scalp. This way there would be only a single scar. The fine scar remaining from the last reduction would be covered by hair transplant grafts, which would be placed directly into the scar tissue.

Flaps and Scalp Lifts

In the 1970s and 1980s, another style of surgical hair restoration involved stretching, lifting and moving around large portions of the hairy part of the scalp to give a full head of hair look in a single procedure. These procedures were performed under general anesthetic, which presented an increased medical risk. There was the risk of visible scars from the large sections of scalp that were moved around, and with some procedures the hair growth direction was backwards, and looked unnatural. There was also increased risk of large patches of tissue death if complications developed, which presented a significant problem in contrast to one or two full size hair transplant grafts failing.

All of these procedures are now only rarely performed, and have been largely replaced by various Follicular Unit Grafting techniques.

12

Follicular Unit Micrografting

By the early 1990s, some hair restoration surgeons had began to regularly cut full size hair transplant grafts into quarters to form minigrafts having three to five hairs each, and entire transplant procedures were done with these minigrafts. Many small round holes were made on the scalp to receive the minigrafts. Minigraft hair transplants had the potential to look more natural than procedures done with larger full-size grafts. However, graft failure rates were initially higher with this new procedure than with full-size grafting.

Improved surgical techniques helped improve small graft survival rates, and soon the procedure evolved further to even smaller micrografts containing only one to three hairs each. This was the beginning of micrograft hair transplants. The method of harvesting donor follicles changed as well. Instead of removing dozens of small pieces of tissue from the back of the scalp, and then cutting these into even smaller pieces, all the donor follicles were removed at one time in the form of adjacent strips of tissue using a multi-bladed scalpel.

Teams of medical assistants then cut 1,000 or more individual micrografts from

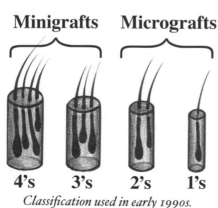

Minigrafts   **Micrografts**

4's   3's   2's   1's

Classification used in early 1990s.

the strips of donor material, using magnifying loupes and glasses. Even with several assistants, micrograft preparation takes several hours, and graft placement takes much longer as well. A micrograft procedure can take a full day, in contrast to a few hours for a full-size graft surgery. But the improved results over full-size grafts and minigrafts were worth the time and effort, and by the early 1990s micrografting became the new standard for surgical hair restoration. A variation of micrografting called follicular unit micrografting continues to be the most popular method of surgical hair restoration in use today.

Micrografting offers numerous advantages over other surgical hair restoration techniques, including full-size graft procedures, scalp reductions, and scalp lifts and flaps. Among the benefits are more natural appearing results, a very short "under construction" period, and each micrograft procedure stands alone, thereby giving both the doctor and patient increased flexibility in addressing the hair loss

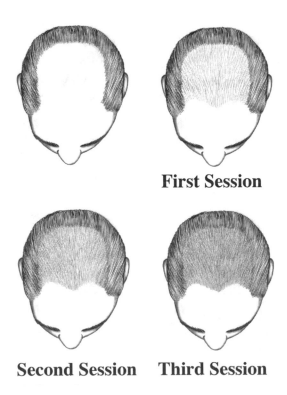

First Session

Second Session   **Third Session**

A series of follicular unit micrograft procedures

condition. Micrografting is a relatively safe procedure, and medical complications or poor cosmetic results are rare.

Achieving more natural appearing results is the primary goal of all elective cosmetic surgical procedures. Micrografts give the surgeon the greatest flexibility in graft placement so that a very natural look can be achieved. Micrografts can be placed between existing hairs, allowing a patient who is just beginning to experience hair loss to increase his or her hair density, and never have that "balding" look. For patients who already have bald areas, a single micrograft procedure will change them from looking like they are losing their hair to an appearance of just having "thin hair." Subsequent procedures can add density, until a "full head of hair" look is achieved.

In addition to appearing more natural than full-size grafts, skillfully placed micrografts can allow for a more effective illusion of having more hair. Colorado hair restoration surgeon Dr. Jim Swinehart considers each graft to be a "visual unit." A single full-size graft having fifteen hairs is like a large tree standing alone in front of a house. The same number of hairs broken up into eight micrografts creates eight "visual units," which can be compared to a quantity of eight bushes spread in front of a house. When the same quantities of hairs are spread out with smaller grafts, they give the appearance of more coverage.

Incisions made for micrograft procedures heal very quickly in comparison to other surgical methods of hair restoration, resulting in a very short "under construction" period. The donor area is closed with a single fine line of sutures, and is well camouflaged by the thicker hair at the back of the head. The recipient sites where the grafts are placed are fine slits made with a miniature surgical blade, and these heal very rapidly. Many micrograft patients return to work a day or two after the procedure, and no one is aware of the work that was done. This is in contrast to the two weeks or longer for healing that is allowed for full size grafts and for incisions made for scalp reductions, lifts, and flaps.

Each micrograft procedure is designed to stand alone, meaning that no additional procedures are required, and that the transplanted hairs will look natural decades in the future even as hair loss progresses. By placing micrografts over the entire balding surface of the scalp, as well as between growing hairs in adjacent areas that will likely lose hair, a skilled surgeon will avoid creating an "island" of dense hair surrounded by thinning hair as hair loss continues years in the future. Micrografting allows for additional procedures to be performed, as the patient desires.

I have had some patients express a desire for the densest possible coverage, anticipating several successive micrografting procedures; however, after a single procedure grows out they are satisfied with their new hair just the way it is. And I've also had patients who initially indicate they want only a single procedure, with just enough coverage to give them some hair on the top or on the back of their heads. Then after a single procedure, they decide to have a few more, in order to achieve maximum density. Micrograft transplants allow for this flexibility.

This is in contrast to the original large grafts (plugs), which required the full series of procedures to fill in the spaces between grafts in order to avoid the "doll's hair" look. With original large plug grafts, if the patient elected not to have all the recommended procedures done, the transplant looked unfinished. Or, if the surgeon miscalculated the degree of future hair loss, an island of dense hair may emerge as the surrounding fringe receded. Micrografting is also employed to enhance previously performed full size graft procedures, as well as to cover scars from scalp reductions, scalp lifts, and flap procedures.

Micrografting is a safe procedure, both medically and cosmetically. In contrast to more elaborate hair restoration techniques such as scalp lifts and scalp flaps, micrografting has a low risk of medical complications. Unlike scalp lift and flap procedures, with micrografting the patient does not receive general anesthesia, and is awake during the entire procedure. General anesthesia alone presents a significant risk of medical complications, and is avoided entirely with micrografting. Other medical complications, while always a possibility with any surgical procedure, are rare with micrografting.

In addition to being medically safe, micrografting is a safe cosmetic procedure as well. A single micrografting procedure almost always produces excellent or very good appearing results, and even a poor micrograft transplant is usually cosmetically acceptable and can be enhanced or corrected. In contrast, more elaborate scalp lift and flap procedures can produce remarkable results with a single surgical session; however, they can also produce disastrous cosmetic results when everything does not go right. Patches of dead scalp tissue and large unsightly scars are examples of complications that have occurred with scalp lifts and flaps.

During the 1990s, many variations of micrografting emerged, with each technique claiming to have special advantages. Examples of variations in micrografting included monografting, megasessions, the use of graft cutting and placement machines, laser hair transplants, and follicular unit micrografting.

MONOGRAFTING

Monografting was the exclusive use of single-hair grafts. It seemed to be a natural evolution from the original full-size pluggy grafts containing up to fifteen hair follicles, to minigrafts having three to five hairs, to micrografts having one to three hairs. The theory was that individually placed hair follicles would give the most natural appearance of all. With this procedure, single-hair grafts were meticulously sculpted to almost bare follicles, and then placed into tiny recipient sites usually made with a surgical needle. Unfortunately, the extensive cutting that was necessary to isolate individual hair follicles resulted in a loss of many donor follicles and a relatively high graft failure rate, and the appearance of the surviving grafts was one of overall fuzziness that did not look natural.

MEGASESSIONS

The first megasessions were another variation of micrografting in which the donor material was cut into 1- and 2- hair grafts, and 2-3,000 or more grafts were placed in a single session. The idea behind megasessions was to solve a patient's hair loss problem in a single surgical procedure. The problem was that each graft had to be trimmed extensively, and the grafts had to be placed very close together. Most of the grafts were 1- and 2-hair grafts, many created from 3-hair grafts. The excessive cutting increased the risk of graft failure from the rough treatment of the thousands of individual grafts. Initially, most responsible hair restoration surgeons avoided placing more than

2,000 grafts in a single session in order to reduce risk to the limited supply of donor follicles. As the techniques improved, the number of grafts per session increased up to 5,000 grafts in one session.

GRAFT CUTTING AND PLACEMENT MACHINES

Because of the length of time and large number of medical assistants needed for micrograft procedures, some early attempts were made to increase efficiency with technology through the use of specialized hair transplantation machines. One device was a "graft-cutting machine" that sectioned the strips of donor tissue into uniform "grafts," in much the same way that a hard-boiled egg slicer would slice an egg into uniform pieces. While this device saved a considerable amount of time and labor, it could cut the tissue without regard to where the hair follicles were located, or their angles of orientation. There was a higher percentage of transection, or cutting of the hair follicles. While some of the sliced hair follicles survived, and on occasion two halves even survived and regrew as two small hair follicles, many more perished, and the device never caught on. Only a few hair transplant surgeons have used graft-cutting machines successfully, and typically with patients having very straight coarse hair. I had the opportunity to see this procedure done by a good hair transplant surgeon using only one assistant. The results were very good. The main drawback to this procedure is that more hairs are lost in the preparation and the patient should have straight hair.

Another attempt at automation was a hand-held graft implantation device that was first loaded with uniformly cut grafts, which the machine then placed into the patient's scalp in much the same manner as a carpenter's nail gun places nails into a roof. The machine pierced the scalp and inserted the graft in one step. In addition to either requiring the aforementioned machine-cut grafts, or very carefully hand-cut grafts, this machine did not seem to actually save much time, and it never became very popular. When used to place the grafts close together, the automatic implanters tend to push out the grafts next to them. More accurate and more densely placed grafts could be accomplished by using a fine blade to make the incision and tedious, meticulous placement using two forceps by experienced placement surgical technicians.

Laser Hair Transplants

Another high-technology micrografting technique was laser hair transplants. The donor material was harvested the same way as for other micrograft procedures, but the recipient sites were made with a laser. The most sophisticated laser hair transplants used computerized scanning devices to make tiny slots for each graft. A problem inherent with using a laser is thermal damage to the cells surrounding the opening made by the laser. Lasers vaporize tissue, and many layers of cells suffer damage from the heat. Grafts placed into laser slots also heal more slowly, and the patient looked "under construction" for a considerably longer time than with other micrografting methods. Some laser transplant surgeons claimed that the recipient slots made by the laser resulted in a more "natural" graft than slits made with steel instruments; however, most surgeons could not perceive a benefit, and certainly not when weighed against the considerable expense of buying or leasing the laser. Laser transplantation allowed for high technology advertising claims, but the procedure never really caught on.

Follicular Unit Micrografting

By the mid 1990s, micrografting evolved into follicular unit micrografting, which is currently considered the state-of-the-art method of hair transplantation. The emphasis of this technique is twofold. The first is maximizing the yield and survival of the limited supply of donor hair follicles throughout every stage of the surgical procedure. The second is on achieving the most natural-looking results possible. Many subtle refinements of the micrografting surgical technique comprise a follicular unit transplant procedure, and combined together these refinements give the best possible results.

The first way in which a follicular unit micrografting procedure may differ from some of the micrografting variations of the past is careful planning to avoid harvesting too many grafts for a single transplant session. Almost every patient wants as much hair density added in as few sessions as possible; however, placing too many micrografts too close together increases the risk of graft failure. Despite the ability to harvest and place many more grafts, a follicular unit micrograft surgeon will choose to do only 1,000 to 2,000 grafts in a single session. The main limitation to the number of grafts per session is the issue of supply and demand. In most patients with extensive balding the donor area is usually much less dense as well as being smaller in size. The patients with very dense donor hair in the back usually are not very bald. I would estimate that only one patient in one hundred would be a candidate for 5,000 grafts, two in a hundred may qualify for 4,000 grafts leaving the majority getting 1,000 to 2,500 per session.

The donor material harvesting method is another refinement that has become a standard part of follicular unit micrografting. In the past, many surgeons used a multi-bladed scalpel to remove the donor tissue from the back of the scalp. All the blades in this surgical instrument were parallel, and were set about three millimeters apart. With a multi-bladed knife, the donor material was removed already cut into long strips, and individual grafts were then more easily cut from the strips. This method caused many hair follicles to be cut by the scalpel blades, and a high percentage of these cut follicles did not survive. Follicular unit surgeons now use a single-blade scalpel to remove the donor tissue from the scalp, and then cut the donor tissue into grafts under high magnification, working to avoid cutting the hair follicles.

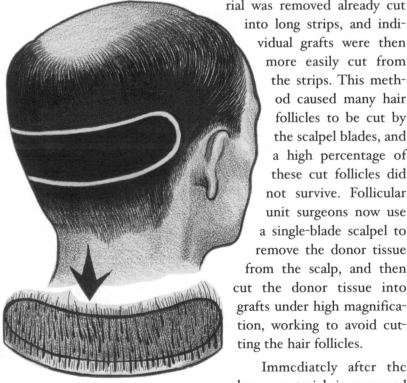

Donor material is removed from the patient.

Immediately after the donor material is removed from the patient, it is immersed in cold saline solution to bring down the temperature of the follicles, and thereby increases graft survival. A few hours can elapse from the time the donor tissue is removed to when a particular hair follicle is placed into the scalp, and keeping the follicles cool and moist helps them survive better during this time. After the grafts are cut they are placed onto surgical pads moistened with saline solution, and these pads are placed into trays that are chilled as well.

The use of stereomicroscopes to cut the donor material into grafts is another standard component of follicular unit micrografting. In the early stages of micrografting, eye loupes and magnifying glasses were commonly used to aid the process of cutting donor tissue into strips and pieces, and eventually into individual grafts; however, a considerable number of hair follicles were cut due to poor visibility even under high magnification.

Stereomicroscopes have separate eyepieces for each eye, which allows for a more three dimensional view of the donor tissue. Stereomicroscopes require additional training for the team of medical assistants who cut the grafts; however, their use results in less follicle transection, meaning they avoid splitting hairs.

Stereomicroscope

To further improve visibility during graft preparation, and to keep the donor tissue cool, I have removed the standard halogen spotlights from all of my graft preparation microscopes and have installed cool fluorescent light panels, which illuminate the grafts from underneath. This lighting technique is called transillumination. Cool fluorescent transillumination helps to make small dormant hair follicles and follicles containing very fine light-colored hairs

109

more visible, further increasing yield. This lighting enhancement also avoids heat damage to the donor tissue that incandescent lighting from the overhead can cause.

The most significant of all micrografting refinements, and the concept that gives the follicular unit procedure its name, is the preservation of the naturally occurring clusters of hair follicles during graft preparation. Transplant surgeons have observed that many hair follicles on the scalp occur in pairs or bundles of three or four follicles, which are called follicular units. Preserving follicular units intact as micrografts reduces the risk of inadvertently cutting follicles occurring close together, which results in grafts growing more viable hairs, and also produces grafts that grow hairs in more natural clusters.

In the early years of micrografting procedures, the hair restoration surgeon would develop a plan for the quantity and size of the hair grafts for a particular procedure. The team of medical assistants may have been instructed to produce 600 single-hair grafts, 500 2-hair grafts, and 400 3-hair grafts for a procedure calling for 1,500 total grafts. The team of medical assistants then cut grafts from the donor tissue according to the surgeon's requirements, and if a certain number of two-hair grafts were needed, clusters of hair follicles were cut apart into two-hair grafts. This inevitably resulted in some accidental cutting and loss of some hair follicles.

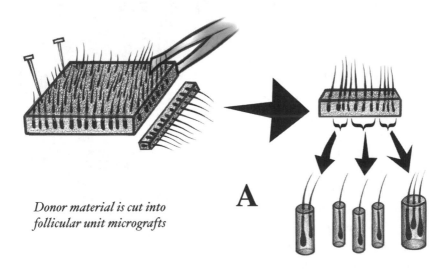

Donor material is cut into follicular unit micrografts

A

With follicular unit transplant procedures, the medical assistants preparing the grafts use their judgment to identify and cut around follicular units, producing grafts containing one, two, or three hairs according to how many follicular units naturally occur in the donor tissue.

Finally, the follicular unit micrografts are placed into tiny slits made in the scalp with a miniature scalpel. I use a blade designed for eye surgery. The slits are made in a slightly irregular manner, to avoid creating a pattern of rows as the grafts begin to grow new hairs. In the early days of micrografting, surgeons were careful to allow adequate space between each graft, and a variation of a grid pattern was used to make recipient sites. With follicular unit micrografting, adequate space is allowed between grafts; however, the grafts are placed in a more random and natural looking manner.

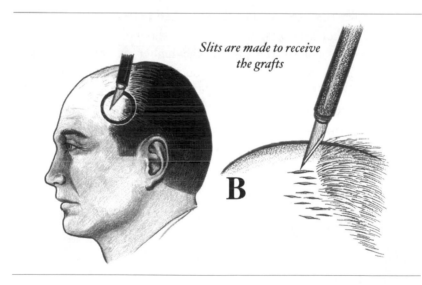

Slits are made to receive the grafts

B

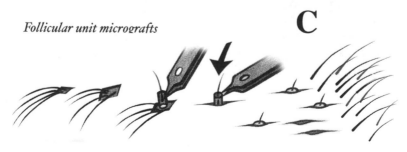

Follicular unit micrografts

C

FOLLICULAR UNIT EXTRACTION (FUE)

This technique of producing follicular unit grafts is possible because of newer, extremely sharp, small sized punches. The technique is similar to the original 4mm full-sized graft technique in that the hair is harvested using a circular punch of 0.75mm to 1.25mm punch (a circular cutting tool similar to a cookie cutter). By using these fine small punches with magnifying loupes, the surgeon can take out intact follicular units ranging from one to three hairs.

When hair transplants were first performed in the 50s and 60s, several studies were conducted to determine the optimum size of a graft using the best punches or trephines of the time. When the grafts were smaller than 3.5 mm in diameter, an increased loss at the periphery of the graft occurred. When the grafts were larger than five mm, loss in the center gave the transplant a donut appearance. Even then we knew the smaller grafts looked better, it was not worth the much higher percentage of hairs lost though transection at the periphery—the smaller the punch, the higher percentage of hairs were lost. Only with the advent of super-sharp small punches has this procedure become more viable, and thus has been more popular and widely used. The FUE method of harvesting grafts is very labor intensive for the surgeon. A much more time consuming process than strip harvesting, it is tiring for both the surgeon and the patient. Not

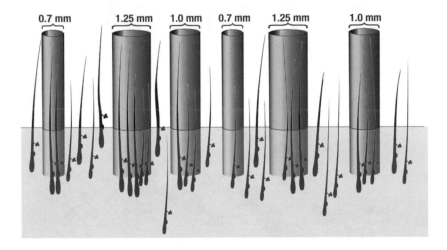

Folliclar Unit Extration

as many grafts can be done at one session and the much larger donor area has to be trimmed short leading to a longer period before looking cosmetically acceptable.

When the procedure was first introduced in 2002, the results I saw were less than impressive. The amount of scarring in the donor area was not acceptable despite claims the area could heal without visible signs that grafts had been harvested. More importantly, there were limitations as to who could have the procedure. Those with curly hair would be rejected because too many of the hairs would be destroyed by cutting through the curved hair follicle. The "Fox Test" was developed and surgeons began to take sample FUE grafts prior to setting up a final surgical appointment. The Fox Test allowed surgeons to evaluate what percentage of follicles would be destroyed on a patient to patient basis. If the percentage was deemed too high for a particular patient, strip harvesting would be recommended. I had an opportunity to observe several procedures done at the DHI Clinic in Athens in September 2004, and I was quite impressed with the lack of scarring in the donor area and the minimal loss of hairs in the harvesting process. Despite these improvements in the FUE technique, most patients would prefer the strip harvesting method due to the more rapid process of moving the hairs and greater comfort during the process.

13

Before, During, and After Surgery

So you're giving serious consideration to micrograft transplant surgery. This chapter explains how to best prepare for a follicular unit micrograft transplant procedure, what it will be like during surgery, and what to expect after the procedure is completed.

The first step after scheduling a procedure is to stop smoking if you are a smoker. Also avoid non-prescription blood-thinning medications and food supplements that may cause excessive bleeding during surgery. A thousand or more tiny incisions are made on the scalp during micrografting surgery, and rapid blood clotting keeps the scalp relatively free of blood during the procedure; this allows the surgeon to work more effectively. Some medications are used during surgery to slightly reduce bleeding; however, it is helpful if the patient takes some additional measures as well. Smoking thins the blood, and certain over-the-counter medications such as aspirin and vitamin supplements such as vitamin E also reduce blood clotting, which can result in extra bleeding during surgery. Excessive bleeding during micrografting does not present a significant medical risk; however, it does slow down the procedure. Avoid aspirin and vitamin E supplements for at least two weeks prior to the surgery.

After scheduling the appointment, prescription medications including pills for pain and antibiotics will be prescribed for use after the surgery. It is best fill to the prescriptions before the scheduled surgery, as you may not feel like waiting in a pharmacy after surgery.

On the day before surgery it is courteous to call the doctor's office or leave a message and confirm your appointment.

The morning of the procedure, shower and wash your hair, but do not use any conditioners or styling products. Use a shampoo without conditioner if possible. If you plan to pay for your surgery with a check, be sure to bring your checkbook. Generally it is good to eat a light meal prior to surgery so that medications provided just before surgery are not taken on an empty stomach, unless advised otherwise by your doctor. Fruit such as grapes, bananas, or apples are good choices. Avoid drinking excessive quantities of liquids, and avoid stimulants such as caffeine and nicotine.

Select layers of comfortable clothes for the surgery. Loose-fitting pants, and shirts with buttons that do not pull over your head are recommended. Jogging outfits with zippered tops are ideal. Operating rooms are frequently heavily air-conditioned and can be very cool, and you will be lying in one place without moving much for several hours. Without some layers of clothing, you may feel chilled. Wear a few layers so that you can adjust what you are wearing easily, and consider bringing a pair of warm socks as well.

Get a ride to the doctor's office, and be sure to arrive on time, or even a little early. After surgery you may still feel a bit drowsy and your reaction time may be slightly impaired. For safety, doctors recommend against driving yourself home after surgery. So it is best to get a ride to the doctor's office, and arrange in advance for a "designated driver" to give you a ride home following the procedure.

Once you've arrived at the office you will put on a surgical top over your other clothing, and will receive medication for the surgery. A tranquilizer pill, and other medication to reduce pain and swelling will be administered at this time. This is also a good time to use the bathroom, even if you think that you don't feel like it. It is inconvenient to have to get up in the middle of surgery to use the toilet.

The surgeon will reconfirm the surgical plan with you, and will mark the area for treatment directly on your scalp. Some photographs will be taken.

You will walk into the room where the surgery will be performed, and lie face down on a special vinyl-covered foam mat designed to keep you comfortable and in the proper position during the procedure.

A narrow strip of hair covering the donor area on the back of your scalp will be trimmed and then the scalp on the back of your head will be cleaned with an antiseptic solution. By this time the pills you took several minutes earlier will start having an effect, and you will be fairly relaxed. The donor area will be numbed with injections of anesthetic medication. There will be a pinprick sting with the first injection, and shortly after that your scalp will feel numb, and it will remain numb for the next several hours.

In addition to the anesthetic, the donor area will be injected with a quantity of saline solution. The saline injections swell the donor site slightly and make harvesting a strip of tissue easier. With a single-blade scalpel, the surgeon will remove the strip of donor tissue. The donor tissue is handed off to a team of medical assistants who begin cutting it into follicular unit micrografts. Meanwhile, the open area on the back of your scalp is closed with sutures. It is a two-step process, with the deepest layer of scalp tissue sewn together with dissolving sutures, followed by the outer layer of skin being closed with removable stitches. Some surgeons use staples to close the donor site; .I have found that while suturing takes a bit longer to perform, my patients find sutures to be more comfortable after surgery. A bandage is placed over the closed wound, and mild pressure is applied to reduce bleeding, usually with a headband.

While the micrograft donor site is being closed, the donor tissue will have been cooled and trimmed to form the first few hundred follicular unit micrografts by the surgeon's team of medical assistants. The medical assistants will use stereomicroscopes to cut around the natural pattern of hair follicle clusters within the donor scalp tissue, as they form grafts containing one, two, or three hairs. Even the largest of these grafts will be smaller than a grain of rice. The graft cutting process will continue for a few hours.

After the donor tissue is harvested and the opening on the back of the scalp is closed, the recipient sites on the front and top your scalp will be prepared. You will most likely change position on the surgical table, and the area that will receive the grafts will be numbed with anesthetic injections. The surgeon will prepare some of the recipient sites for the grafts. I use a miniature surgical blade that was originally designed for eye surgery to make the tiny slits that will receive the follicular unit micrografts. Great care is taken in placing and angling the recipient sites to assure that the grafts will grow out in a natural direction and without a detectable pattern. Some grafts will be between existing growing hairs, and great care is taken to avoid damage to existing hair follicles while assuring adequate space between each graft.

The follicular unit micrografts are placed into the recipient sites according to the surgical plan. Typically single-hair grafts are used to create a hairline, and multi-hair grafts are used to fill in the top and back areas, where they add greater hair density. As the first hundred recipient sites are filled with grafts, the surgeon will prepare additional sites. Meanwhile the medical assistants are continuing to cut more follicular unit micrografts. Placing the individual grafts may take two to three hours, depending upon the quantity of grafts prepared. During this time, it is common for the patient to doze off, and occasionally reawaken. Eventually all the grafts are placed into recipient sites, and the surgery is completed.

After placing all of the grafts, your scalp is gently cleaned, so that the grafts are barely visible. Most of my patients leave the office without any bandages. Typically you will be given some water and something to eat after surgery. You will also be given some medications to reduce discomfort and swelling after the local anesthetic wears off. More photographs will be taken. If you need to call for a ride home, this is a good time to make that call. Before leaving, you will pay for your surgery. The staff will ask you questions and observe you, for your own safety, to assure that you are okay to leave.

At home you should avoid vigorous activity and excessive exposure to the sun, which could injure the grafts. Once you are home you may want to take a prescription pain pill, primarily to reduce discomfort from the donor area, which may feel a bit "tight." The pain medication will also help you rest more comfortably. Many patients find that the discomfort following surgery is minor and take some ibuprofen; some patients choose not to take any pain medications at all.

Follow the instructions for care and cleaning your scalp during the healing period which will last about a week. Very gentle shampooing helps to remove traces of blood crusts after the first day, and keeps the scalp clean. Within a few days the grafts will heal so well that they will be just about invisible, especially if they were placed between existing hairs. You will be applying an antibiotic ointment every day to keep the new grafts moist, and to help avoid infections. You will also take prescription antibiotic capsules to further reduce the risk of infections. If any unusual complications occur, including excessive swelling, redness, bumps, or bleeding, contact the office and be prepared to go in that day. Most micrograft patients choose to go back to work one or two days after surgery.

After about a week, you will return to the surgeon's office for the removal of sutures at the donor site. This takes only a couple of minutes and is painless. The surgeon will inspect your scalp to assure that everything is healing well and will take more pictures. During your visit, you may meet other prospective patients in the office who will ask you about your micrografting experience.

Within a week the transplanted hair follicles will appear to be growing new hairs. These are the hairs that they had been growing before they were transplanted.

Usually these old hairs fall out as the transplanted follicles go into the telogen or resting stage after transplantation. Minoxidil lotion can be used to help minimize the shock to the new hair follicles; loss of the donor hairs within the first week is perfectly normal. Immediately after surgery the transplanted grafts will begin to develop new connections to the blood supply. Once the new blood supply is fully established, they will begin to grow new hairs on a permanent basis. This usually takes four to six months.

The new hairs will grow at the rate of about one-half inch a month, just as all the other hairs on your head grow. After about four to six months the transplanted follicles will have grown out hairs long enough to begin contributing some additional density to your hair. The transplanted follicles will continue growing new hairs for as long as the hair follicles still on the back of your head keep growing new hairs.

If you want additional hair density, after six to nine months, you are ready for another micrograft procedure. Some patients are satisfied with a single follicular unit micrografting procedure, and others choose to have additional procedures to add thickness. Additional procedures can be done six to nine months apart, which allows the new grafts adequate time to heal, and produce visible hairs. The new grafts are then placed between the existing hairs, regardless of whether the existing hairs were naturally occurring or transplanted.

14

Marco's Story

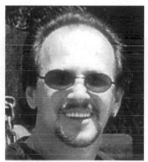

Marco Before Surgery, in 1999

Marco of San Francisco is a renowned professional hairstylist, who currently makes "hair-cutting house calls" by appointment only, and is the author of the book, *It'll Grow Back: How To Communicate With Your Hairstylist Before It's Too Late.* He graduated from Wilfred Academy Beauty School in 1965 and from Robert Fiance Advanced Hairstyling in 1966. He has worked on the East Coast and in Los Angeles, where he was associated with the *Jon Peters* and *She and He* salons. Marco's clients have included business executives, Hollywood actors and actresses, and rock stars. He opened his own salon, The Galerie, in San Francisco in 1981. Marco's style is to cut hair so that people look good, not so that haircuts look good.

Like many men, Marco began losing his hair. The thinning was hardly noticeable at first, but after several years went by his condition became increasingly difficult to hide, especially from himself. A few years after that Marco's hair loss began to affect his self-image, and his business. Finally, in May 2000, Marco decided to do something about his own hair loss.

This is Marco's story, told in his own words:

121

Finally Facing the Truth

It's 3 A.M.

The TV had been turned off, the computer shut down, and even the crickets were quietly sleeping. In the cozy dark of the night, the children gently stirred in happy dreams, and the dog and cat snoozed side by side.

Gentle smiles graced every sleeping face in the world. Everyone, that is, except me.

From deep, deep down in the downstairs bathroom, a faint but ominous light hinted that all was not well behind the tightly locked door. A long, low muffled moan from within betrayed my deepest fears:

"Ohhhhhh Nooooooo!"

It wasn't supposed to be like this. Here I was, a grown adult man staring in the mirror at three in the morning when I should have been sound asleep, resting calmly for my busy day to come. Up until now, I had actually managed to forget all about my problem—forget and go on just like nothing was wrong. That was until a few weeks ago, at the airport, picking up my five-year-old daughter from a visit to her grandparents. As I bent down to grab her pink suitcase off the crowded carousel I heard the fateful words that rang in my ears ever since:

"That's my dad! *The bald guy!*"

The bald guy! The bald guy! My own daughter, for goodness sakes! Hadn't I been a good father? Hadn't I taken her to Disneyland this spring? What unspeakable deed had I done to deserve such demeaning abuse—in public? I would accept any lack of fatherly devotion as an explanation for my daughter's totally inappropriate and disrespectful comment rather than—rather than the *truth*.

And then there was last week at that party.... Hey, I may have moved into the successful, married-with-child two-car family set, but I will always be hip. I was hip when I was fourteen playing the sexy, seductive lover in the high school production of "Bye Bye Birdie." I was hip and young and single, living in the 70s. And I still know how to keep a party moving, serving exactly the right wine, telling the funniest jokes, just being me. But last week I could have exited a party by way of the balcony when I heard those words again. Two young women were having a conversation, and I distinctly overheard one remark:

"But he is so cute for a *balding guy!*"

Please, not you too! What had I done to deserve such treatment? The bald guy! Was it a bad year for the merlot? Did I say something to offend you? It had to be some mistake!

You see: the bald guy was someone else. Someone who wore orange and turquoise plaid suits and had glasses as thick as crystal balls held up with masking tape.

Back in the downstairs bathroom, I begged; *"Please, mirror, please,"* as I angled my wife's compact to get a clear view of the back of my head in the bathroom sink mirror, *"say it ain't so!"*

But the wicked mirror only confirmed my worst fears—a shiny, expanding patch of flesh at the top of my head was devouring my remaining hair like an intergalactic blob of plasmic goo. It looked like I was wearing a skin-tight yarmulke made of orange Mylar. I, the legendary hair stylist, the renowned Marco of San Francisco who lived, breathed and ate hair, was indeed going bald! I, who had combed, cut, permed, tinted and styled world leaders and rock stars, was losing my greatest natural asset. And what was worse, the baldness pattern my head displayed was distorting my features in a very, very unflattering way.

IT'S YOUR HEAD

Actually, some people can do "bald" quite well. Take, for example, the gentleman in the top hat, the astronaut with the shaved skull, or the artist with the beret and goatee. These men not only look OK without hair, they actually look their best in a bare head.

How you wear your hair really does affect your features, both from the front (what you see in the mirror), and from the side and back (what everybody else sees). And, because your features are unique, it is important to wear your hair in a way that complements your features in a flattering way. That is why, while many cuts may seem attractive, they are actually not designed for every face. For

123

example, misjudged bangs can turn a woman with a slightly angular head into a square-jawed quarterback for the Oakland Raiders.

Over years of styling hair, I developed quite a science for determining how hair affects various features. How, for example, the perception of the shape and size of your head is directly determined by hairstyle. You can buy the most expensive, trendy cut in town, but if it short-changes your natural curves and angles, you are likely to look awkward.

And just like a crew cut, a ponytail or sideburns, bald dramatically affects your features, for better or for worse. In my case, and that of many men, bald definitely affected us for the worse. Balding caused my oval face to elongate into an oblong head—the face I had counted on my entire life left and was replaced by this stranger sitting on my shoulders.

The image I have for myself is smart, sexy, confident and successful. In fact, the self-confidence I need to project is so great that it affects my audience—from an auditorium full of colleagues at a conference, to a one-on-one with a new client—so that they feel comfortable and secure with my abilities. As a hair stylist myself, I need to inspire my clients by showing them that I have the wherewithal to overcome hair loss and project a look that demonstrates that I really know my business.

Bald just did not fit my personality, period. It did not fit my body. It did not fit my career. So on many nights I found myself locked in the downstairs bathroom asking God, "Why me? Why did you give me this unwanted permanent haircut? I don't remember asking you for a style suggestion."

It didn't fit, it had no mercy, and I didn't want it.

YOU DON'T HAVE TO BE BALD!

The answer was really terribly, terribly simple. There have been huge advances in hair loss treatment in recent years, and hair transplant surgery delivers the greatest promise of them all:

With hair transplant surgery you will be able to once again grow and maintain your own hair, growing out of your own head. Your hair loss will be a forgotten thing of the past.

Aaaah, it sounds like the promise that is too good to be true. But how does one find out for himself before committing to an expensive and life-altering treatment? Researching the hair-transplant field is a lot trickier than researching the new car market, and that's exactly what I've been doing for the last five years. As a professional stylist and as a man suffering from hair loss, I've met with just about every hair-transplant specialist on the West Coast. I want to know how these doctors approach their clients, the surgical procedures and, most of all, the results.

Well the truth is that as a professional stylist I see hundreds of men and cut their hair. I've seen some really bad transplant jobs out there. Do you know what happens when you get the wrong job? It can look like trees are sprouting all over your head. In the past, some surgeons grafted those little follicles in ten or twelve at a time, the same way those hairs are grouped on the head of my daughter's Barbie dolls. Instead of a nice wavy head of corn silk, you end up with dreadful little clumps bursting up in a crosshatched pattern all over your skull.

And even worse, in some cases those follicles can die after transplantation. If you thought anything could be worse than going bald, imagine your own head covered with little scars, looking like tracks. It looks like a truck ran over your poor, already-bald head.

With a shudder, I considered how intimate I would become with my mirror and our 3 A.M. talks, if there were no an alternative to the potential Frankenstein-effect of the hair-transplant.

But bad hair transplants are now pretty rare. I see a lot more excellent hair transplant jobs. Some transplants make guys look phenomenal! Not only is it impossible to detect the grafts, but the shape, the style, the thickness is just right for them, and blends perfectly into their natural hair and features. These guys have gotten back the original shape of their heads, and the full, natural, free feeling of their own hair.

What these guys have that I want is follicular unit micrografts. Follicular unit micrograft hair-transplantation is an art by which naturally-occurring clusters of hair follicles are carefully seeded into your scalp so that their thickness, direction and shape precisely mimics your own natural hair. I did my research, and I selected Dr. Peter Panagotacos to do my hair.

Dr. Panagotacos had performed tens of thousands of successful micrograft transplants, transforming men all over the world from that bald guy into that successful leader, artist, father, teacher, actor, sexy, happy, confident guy.

Within a couple of weeks, I could make an appointment, have the surgery, and walk into life with the confidence and stature of a man who has been given a new lease on life. No problem, right?

But Did You Consider

How long has it been since you've had a full head of hair? For me it's been about ten solid years since I gave in to the fact that my hair loss was inevitable—but a good fifteen or twenty years if you count the denial associated with gradual thinning. As a stylist I know that for most men undergoing a hair transplant, it's been as many as twenty years since you've given up on the mousse, donated the bristle-brush to the dog, and taken to washing your remaining fuzz with Soft-soap, hot water or toothpaste. The last real haircut you bothered to get was for a Grateful Dead concert, and even then you spent most of the show envying the hair on some of those aging musicians.

Your life, your career and your schedule are probably fundamentally different than they were twenty years ago. First, you are going to have to consider how to take care of your new hair. Remember that aisle at the supermarket with shampoo and brushes and all kinds of gels and mousse? Well, you're not only going to have to purchase the appropriate products for your hair, but you're also going to have to relearn how to use them.

"Easy," you say? Well, just consider how much time you took in your twenties to blow-dry and style your hair every day. An hour? And that little comb sticking out of your back pocket that came out every time a girl walked by, or every time you passed a mirror? Where did you get all that time? How will you fit your hair care into your Palm Pilot?

And you are going to have to decide what your new head of hair is going to look like. What was that style you wore to the Grateful Dead or to the disco? Would it be appropriate for the boardroom? Client meetings? Presentations? Do you simply want to display your ability to outwit Mother Nature, or do you have an inner cool—a personal confidence—you want to awaken and leverage with your new hair? For the past fifteen years or so, the wicked fates have controlled your look, but now you can be back in the driver's seat. Which features are you going to accentuate? Which ones will you soften? What is the combination that spells success for your personal vision?

Once again, a professional hair stylist is going to be a key player in your life. And to help you move forward and express a look that enhances your vision, it is crucial to create your new style from a set of criteria that includes your daily schedule, career and goals, as well as the physical construction of your face. As a professional hair stylist I firmly believe that your hair care professional should be your partner in creating the look that's right for you. However, since not all stylists take that approach, you are going to need a set of communication tools to ensure that you get your message across and end up getting the most from your new hair.

As I looked in the mirror, I was convinced that the new me would be sexy rather than conservative, carry the attitude of a seasoned professional, and give me the confidence to perform better. My face will not be framed by baldness, or by the carefree hair of a twenty-year-old, but by the mature, commanding head of hair I was meant to have at this point in my life. *Look out life! Marco of San Francisco shall reign again!*

GOING FROM BALD TO BOLD

I heaved a sigh of relief. The quest was at its end. Or so I thought. A successful transplant process is really much, much more than just checking in and out of a doctor's office for surgery, and then driving off in your convertible. Undergoing the consultations, surgery, and waking up to the possibilities of a new head of hair is a complex conversation you need to have with yourself, your hair-transplant doctor, and your stylist. Using myself as a guinea pig, I am going to give you a first-hand account in the following pages of just what to expect, what to watch out for and plan for as you go from bald to bold.

First there is the interview. How are you going to communicate your vision to the doctor? This isn't a haircut where you can afford to take a chance, and then re-do it three months later if it didn't work out. And how comfortable would the doctor make me? What could I do to prepare? Certainly not belting back a stiff drink. That one-hour interview would really affect how I looked for the rest of my life.

Then there is the operation itself. I've heard it's not all that bad, but I just don't like hospitals or doctor's offices, or the idea of wearing a surgical mask on the top of my head. What would I do to keep the anticipation from dominating the rest of my life?

And as the new hair grows in, would it be like spring flowers, where every day there is a bit more difference, more growth? Would I find myself staring at my new hair for hours in the bathroom mirror at 3:00 A.M., but unwilling to let anyone else see? They say that after a week you can't even tell the difference any more, but when would I be satisfied?

And what about "The Big Day?" How would my family react? My colleagues? Would I blush when I went in to work, would people know? Would curious children want to run their fingers through it in fascination? How about sexy women? How about my wife?

The road ahead is long, and it's very important that I make the right decisions at each step of the way, but now I have a vision. A vision of my personal successes, of my daughter being proud of her good-looking dad, of no more 3:00 A.M. talks with the mirror, and of a confident, sexy, younger looking me.

THE RESULTS ARE IN!

I lay in bed and drowsily smiled. The world blurred in and out of existence as the effects of Dr. Panagotacos' three-pill 'cocktail' gradually began to recede. Not six hours ago I had been on the operating table with Dr. Panagotacos and three more-than-capable nurses having the back of my head cut and all the hairs therein—3,800 of them—transplanted on the top of my head. Wow, I'd finally done it, after all these years of telling myself I could. "You see, God," I thought, "I always knew there would be a way. And now, I have just one thing to ask. *And that is—Did I have won-ton today?*"

WON-TON?

Just how strong was that so-called "cocktail"? Where was the merciless scalp pain I had received so many warnings about? Shouldn't I be running back and forth to the bathroom to count each individual new hair, charting its hour-to-hour growth progress?

Truth be known, long after that little cocktail had worn off, my memory of the day long surgery revolved around the question of whether or not I had hallucinated eating a really yummy bowl of Chinese soup with Dr. Panagotacos—smack dab in the middle of my hair transplant surgery.

Not that hair transplant surgery is quite as easy as eating a bowl of soup. For example, the night before my operation, I had a lot more than the next day's lunch on my mind.

The butterflies started in my stomach the night before. We've all had butterflies before a trip to the doctor, and some of us before a trip to the barber, but the night-before-the-hair-transplant butterflies are unique. They are every kind of butterfly you've ever had combined. Not only would my outward appearance be irreversibly altered; not only was the transplant the culmination of years of research and personal visioning: but some people I had been talking to had suggested that a hair transplant might involve PAIN.

About friends who want to tell you all kinds of stories about transplants and pain—don't listen to 'em. I sure wish I hadn't. There are lots of folks out there who will tell you all kinds of crazy things about post-transplant pain—everything from itchiness to blood squirting out of the tops of their heads. If you try hard enough, you'll find someone with just the right horror story to send you into nightmares for weeks before your transplant.

I don't know if these so-called friends are some new breed of super-wimps or if they just drum up these tales to watch you squirm, but take it from me—you don't need the advice. You're going to be just fine.

The actual process of having a transplant is one of the most relaxed, worry-free, painless stages of life's hair experience. It's done on-site in a doctor's office and usually takes about six to eight hours— you come in at 8:00 A.M., and by 4:00 P.M. you're on your way home. It's like going to work, but instead of sitting at an ergonomically unsound desk worrying about next quarter's figures, you spend the day on a special surgical chair, stoned out of your mind, surrounded by great-looking nurses.

"Good morning, Marco," the nurses said, when I walked into Dr. Panagotacos' office on that Monday morning in May. I thought they were going to ask me whether I'd prefer merlot or Chablis. By the time Dr. Panagotacos sat down with me, I was starting to feel pretty comfortable. They asked me some standard questions, showed me some pictures, made a few jokes and then the process got under way. First, they gave me a three-pill "cocktail." Now I'm not saying what's in that cocktail, nor am I even sure I fully know myself, but when that kicked in, every bit of remaining fear vanished. They could have cut my foot off and I wouldn't care.

"Ahoy there, Doctor!" I thundered, "I reckon I'll swim over to that table about now!"

"So you're ready to begin the hair transplant, Marco?" the nearest nurse inquired.

"Nurse," I said, "I'm going scuba diving, and I wonder if you'd come with me to my kingdom under the sea?"

At this point I'd like to note that while the operation itself is completely painless, men may experience considerable pain if their wives ever hear what they said while under the influence of "the cocktail." In my own defense, I didn't even recognize the nurse I had propositioned the next time I walked into the office.

The nurse then proceeded to completely numb the back of my scalp with the same kind of injections a dentist uses. Under the influence of "the cocktail" all I felt was the lightest pressure—maybe as if I had on a hat that was one size too tight.

The next part of the operation requires the removal of the donor hairs, which is an inch wide strip of scalp. The doctor removes the strip from the hair-rich region on the back of your head where you'll never miss it. It's from that strip of scalp that the hairs are extracted for transplanting into your cap. The skin is quickly stitched back together while the nurses begin working vigorously under the microscopes to remove individual follicular units for transplant.

When people talk about "pain," the donor area is usually the part of the procedure they are referring to. In my case, and in most cases, there will be a slight feeling of tightness or maybe an itching feeling for about a week where the skin is stitched back together. This very superficial discomfort entirely disappeared the second the nurses took the stitches out a week after the surgery. The scar, if noticeable at all, is and unobtrusive fine line, and completely hidden by your natural hair.

As the nurses removed the 3,800 or so hairs from the extracted skin and turn them into little follicular unit grafts, Dr. Panagotacos expertly placed them up on my top. The mark of an expert is in the subtle attention to detail, and Dr. Panagotacos definitely lived up to my expectations. First, those grafts were individually placed, avoiding the "hair-forest effect".

Second, they were placed in a shape that was carefully created to mimic a natural hairline for a man my age, rather than the hairline of a teenager (although I admit I'd still like to see what I'd look like with the hairline of my early twenties)

Third, and in my opinion the most impressive, the individual grafts were placed at angles to mimic natural cowlicks, waves and parts. That means that instead of 3,800 hairs growing pell-mell out the top of my head like a punk rock zombie, my hair will have shape and character, just like the natural hair we are born with.

Although I'm sure I had an incredible won-ton meal somewhere during that procedure, the next thing I remembered was that beautiful and tolerant nurse gently shaking me awake. I guess I dozed off during surgery. Without moving, I opened my left eye and carefully looked about for any lingering pain that might have been waiting at the threshold of consciousness, but none was there. So I opened both eyes and put my feet on the ground. To my relief, I felt no pain. Nothing but the receding silliness of the remaining pills.

"Dangkoo, Dott-or," I attempted groggily. "Dat wuzzent too bad."

"Thank YOU, Marco," the staff proudly trilled. "You make sure and get some rest…"

"Wazabbout da won-ton?" I asked, flashing on a memory of the delicious mystery meal.

"Oh—so long to you, too!"

And then, in the passenger seat of my friend's BMW, I was headed home in rush hour traffic, to begin a new life. I chuckled when, in the rear-view mirror, I caught a glimpse of the peach fuzz growing out of the top of my head in a style that was pleasantly similar to the buzz cuts that Tony the Barber used to give me in New Jersey when I was eight or nine.

When you get home from your transplant, make sure you come home to exactly the environment in which you need to recover. For me that meant sending my daughter over to her friend's for the night, and stocking the refrigerator with pasta, chicken soup and a variety of foods I'd prepared in advance. I rented twenty-four hours worth of the latest releases at the local video store, and bought two gallons of coffee ice cream with walnuts. Dr. Panagotacos had given me another "pill cocktail" to get me through the night, along with about eight pain pills to subdue any residual discomfort. My wife Janet had to work late, so the house was completely empty, leaving me nothing to do but take another "pill cocktail" and sleep it off.

That bed felt like the mist of heaven as I smiled myself into a deep, healing sleep.

Later on, when Janet did come in I was barely able to move my eyelids.

"Oh Marco," she breathed softly, "You've done it! You've finally realized your dream and conquered your hair loss. You must feel wonderful!"

"Wuzzza wuzza won-ton?" I mumbled.

Over the next few weeks I made some of the most profound discoveries about the hair growth process of my entire career as a stylist. Life returned more or less to normal over the next few days. My daughter came home, I returned the videos, got tired of pizza for every meal, and resumed everyday life. Two days after the procedure I returned to light duty as a stylist, performing cuts. Although I had eight pain pills in the medicine cabinet I never felt the need to take any of them (although every single client to whom I mentioned the pills made a ploy, an offer, or a plea for even one of the happy capsules). For me the pain had been greatly overestimated, and in hindsight seemed almost like a trivial worry.

The most important thing to remember during that first week is to keep using the antibiotic ointment they give you. There are no reasons for taking any chances with that new crop of hair of yours, so grease yourself up like a championship engine and you'll be all right.

Dr. Panagotacos believes in providing those new little hairs with plenty of fertilizer. Fertilizer for your head is called Rogaine. Right after those stitches come out, you start spraying it on. Rogaine is credited with growing hair on totally barren heads, so imagine what it can do for those 3,800 or so new seedlings. Another supplement Dr. Panagotacos recommends is Propecia. Propecia is a drug that prevents hair loss, and after the stitches are out, one tablet a day helps you keep the hair you have.

In addition to the antibiotic ointment, the Rogaine, and the Propecia, I also bought a beret in case the new hair grew in funny. But it didn't grow in funny at all. What a hair transplant does that isn't so funny, is that it all falls out after the first few weeks. It takes four to six months for the transplanted hair follicles to begin to grow new hairs on a permanent basis.

A week after I had the transplant, friends doubted whether I had undergone the procedure at all. I couldn't blame them either—all the grafts had healed so well, and the scar at the back of my neck had fused so quickly that there was no physical evidence that I had ever been to Dr. Panagotacos and had a transplant.

Well, anything worthwhile is worth waiting for, and at that point I'd been bald or balding for almost two decades so a few more months seemed reasonable, considering the payoff at the end. I donated the beret to my daughter—she, in turn, placed the thing on her pet stuffed elephant.

WHAT TO EXPECT

Four to six months of just being me. Just being plain old Marco Schatzman with a shiny flesh-colored yarmulke on top of my head. No immediate gratification, no super powers.

Which brings me to the most important point of this chapter. A hair transplant is a cosmetic change, and the appearance of new growth on your head is not automatically going to make you a better person or solve any other problems.

As I began the long four to six month wait for the new hair to emerge, I became more and more certain that while a new "look" was developing beneath my scalp, what I did with that hair was going to be entirely up to me. Nothing is more critical to a successful hair transplant than the patient being very clear on his vision of personal success, and how hair will help him achieve that.

In my line of business, first impressions are very important, and I did not like presenting myself to the world as a bald person. When I would meet a new client or associate, I always had the feeling that I would have communicated better, had more confidence, and been less distracted, if it weren't for the lingering feeling that I did not look the best I possibly could.

What could 3,800 hairs do that I couldn't do on my own? When you are feeling good—when you know you've got nothing to worry about—people around you can't help but be affected by your positive attitude. When I'm with someone, whether a client or a friend, I want to be one hundred percent there. With the bald spot, I'd find myself getting distracted thinking that I wasn't looking my best. But now without those worries, I am going to radiate the kind of confidence that will have everyone in the room feeling upbeat. People might never know what changed about Marco (although I'd find no discomfort telling them all about my transplants), but they definitely were going to be totally jazzed about me. They were going to be turned on to me because I was turned on to me.

Although I hate to say it, what with my work, my daughter's various lessons, and my wife's kind of nutty schedule, I'd all but forgotten about my transplant over the summer. Two months after the procedure, the first little sprouts started peeking out from my scalp. Every day I felt growth on the top of my head—rapid growth. It was like one of those movies where they speed up time and you get to watch a flower grow and bloom in a matter of minutes. I kept putting my hand up to my head to see what had landed there. The final results will be in by November when I will be celebrating my fifty-second birthday—the first hairy birthday in almost fifteen years of tucking, folding and compensating to cover that bald spot.

A good surgeon knows you can add hair to a bald area with transplants, but it's difficult to remove it later without visible scars. For that reason, it's best not to get hair transplanted unnaturally low on your forehead (like you had it as a teenager). Remember, your new hair will have to work for you in the boardroom, at presentations, as well as in social settings.

Dr. Panagotacos gave me the hairline of a forty to fifty-year-old man, off the forehead and with a slight peak at the center. I think that's a pretty good look for a CEO, but I decided I'm going to have him lower my hairline to the thirty-five-year-old mark next time I go in. In any case, I was glad to have the option to go further, guided by the expert opinion of Dr. Panagotacos regarding the hairline that would be appropriate for me.

In the meantime, thoughts about my hair turned to how I would style it, how my face would look as a soft, pleasing oval, and how happy I would be to shave off the compensating beard that had adorned my face ever since I had admitted defeat many years ago.

I picked up the phone and called Dr. Panagotacos to discuss the next chapter of my hair growth.

He asked if there was any pain? "No," I replied.

I told him they all fell out a few weeks after the procedure. "Right on time!" he chuckled.

And then I asked him the question that had really been on my mind. "Dr. Panagotacos," I started, "I have this, uh, memory, and I'm not sure if it was real or a hallucination. But I have the strangest feeling that, well, in the middle of the surgery you and I were having won-ton soup."

Apparently we were. "I always order lunch for my patients," Dr. Panagotacos replied. "Nourishment is very important during a transplant."

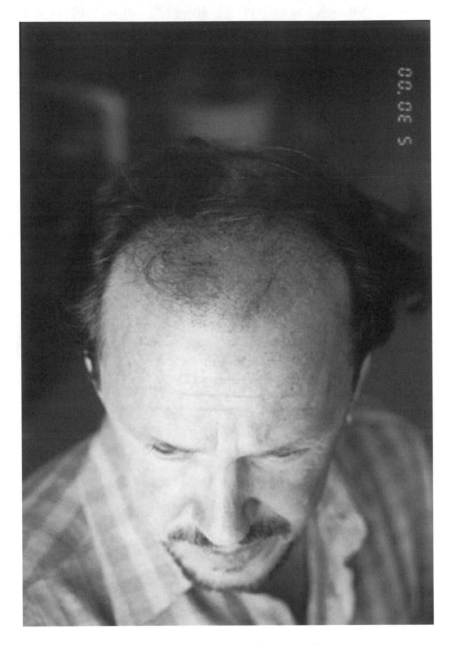

Chapter Ten

Marco in May 2000 with 2000 grafts

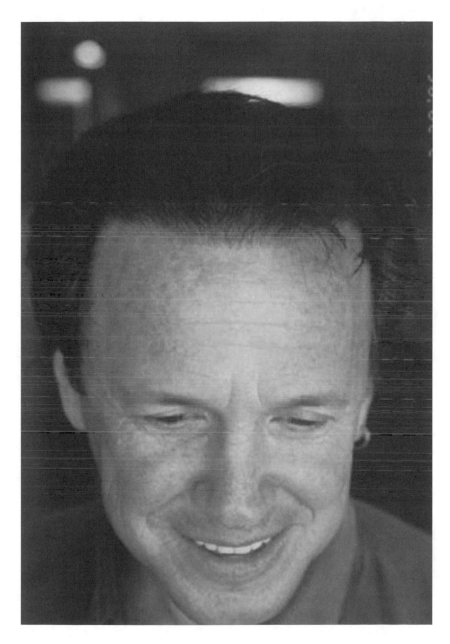

Marco in 2005

15

"Ask the Expert"

I am often asked hair-related questions by medical students when I lecture at hospitals, from other dermatologists when I give presentations at American Academy of Dermatology meetings, and from patients who schedule appointments at either of my San Francisco dermatology practice offices.

I also answers questions from men and women of all ages who contact me through my web site (www.hairdoc.com), or from various on-line chat groups, and "answer" web sites such as allexperts.com.

The following are some examples of some typical, and some not-so-typical, hair loss and hair growth questions, and my answers. Similar questions have been grouped together, and there has been some editing for clarity.

Many young men contact me about their hair loss. Often they are terrified, and some of their attempts to address their "problem" reveal the impact that hair loss at an early age is having on their lives:

QUESTION FROM A 15-YEAR-OLD FEMALE:

I have been pulling my hair out for a while now. I would give anything to get it to grow back! Please help me! Are there any pills or medications I can take that will make my hair grow faster? Please, I am only fifteen-years-old! It's hard to wake up every morning and try to cover up all my disgusting bald spots on my head! I can't even wear my hair down anymore! Please.... Give me some advice! Anything!!!

ANSWER:

Your condition is more complicated than an answer by e-mail can do justice. It is important to determine the reason you are pulling your hair. Start by seeing a dermatologist, to determine if you have a medical condition that needs treatment, and perhaps to talk about other possible causes. You may have issues that are troubling you, and you may be referred to another professional whom you can talk with more easily than the dermatologist, or your parents. Often hair-pulling behavior is a temporary condition, and with some therapy it may clear up quickly.

QUESTION FROM AN 18-YEAR-OLD FEMALE:

Recently I've been experiencing an abnormal amount of hair loss. When I brush my hair, or even just pull on it, hair comes out. There's no history of this in my family, and I'm on no medication, and I'm not sick, except for having a really bad cold for the past three weeks. I'm really worried. Do you know of anything that could cause this?

ANSWER:

A really bad cold can cause actively growing hair follicles to shift into the resting phase, and a few weeks to a couple of months later the hairs in those follicles can start to shed. Normally, about ninety percent of the hair follicles are in the growing phase, and about fifty to 100 hairs are shed each day from other hair follicles that are in the regression and resting phases. A severe stress can increase the percentage of hairs going into the resting phase, and as a result increase the amount of hairs being shed each day, sometimes quite dramatically. You may consider seeing a dermatologist to make sure the loss is not due to some other cause, such as iron deficiency anemia. If your hair loss is due to stress from the bad cold, Rogaine applied every day for a few months can help reduce the shedding until the hair follicles go back to their normal growth cycle.

QUESTION FROM AN 18-YEAR-OLD FEMALE:

During the last two years I have been going through a stage where I had very crazy hair. I dyed my hair many times and had gravity-defying hairstyles. I think my hair was in total stress, because now I notice that my hair is a lot thinner. I remember when I was styling my hair before, I had hair falling off, but I didn't think much of it because I had lots of hair. I believe it is just hair breakage, because when I saw my hair coming off, I didn't see the "bulb" or anything. I'll stop mistreating my hair now, and I hope it will grow back. It should because all the women in my family have lots of hair. Even my grandmother, she has lots of hair. But my brother and dad do suffer from hair loss. Is there a chance I might be suffering from that too?? You don't think I am losing hair permanently do you? I am still very young and I don't want to become bald when I am thirty. How can I stop this from happening?

ANSWER:

From your description of the situation I do not think you are suffering from permanent hair loss. Women do inherit a tendency for pattern hair loss, just as men do; however, many of these women do not exhibit hair loss or even hair thinning. When women with genetic programming for hair loss do start losing hair, they usually suffer a generalized thinning of hair late in life, especially on the top of their heads, rather than developing completely hairless bald spots. It is possible to accelerate the appearance of inherited pattern hair loss by repeatedly pulling hairs from the hair follicles with tight braids and other hair styling techniques that pull on the hairs. Each time a hair shaft is pulled from the follicle, the follicle starts a new growth cycle, which if the hair was not pulled out, may not have happened for five or more years. Dermatologists call this type of hair loss traction alopecia. I believe that hair follicles have a limited number of growth cycles in them, and then they stop growing new hairs. Each time a hair is pulled out from a hair follicle before it was ready to be shed, the hair follicle is one step closer to not growing any new hair. This is why plucking eyebrow hairs or repeatedly having waxing treatments to pull out unwanted hairs can eventually reduce hair growth.

But it is more likely that your hair loss involves the hair shaft, and not the hair follicles where the hair grows from. The hair shaft is made of dead cells that are the visible hair strands that we generally think of as "hair." Your hair has probably suffered repeated exposure to chemicals in hair dyes and perhaps excessive heat from styling techniques that have weakened the hair shafts and caused increased breakage. This is the easiest hair loss problem to treat: simply stop doing the things that damage the hair shafts, and the condition will correct itself as the hair grows out. Keep in mind that hair only grows about one half inch per month, so it may take several months for you to notice an improvement.

QUESTION FROM A 20-YEAR-OLD FEMALE:

I am a black female and I am going bald in the center of my head. Sometimes it itches really bad and it is sore. Can you please give me some advice about my hair loss?

ANSWER:

The type of baldness you are describing really needs to be examined for you to receive proper advice. You may have a bacterial or fungal infection that may respond well to prescription medication. It is possible this condition could have been triggered by "Hot Comb" treatments that can irritate the hair follicles and increase the risk of infection. If the condition continues without treatment it may cause permanent scarring in the affected area, and this could include a permanent bald spot. I recommend that you schedule an appointment with a dermatologist for an examination and treatment.

QUESTION FROM A 24-YEAR-OLD FEMALE:

I have recently started losing my hair and had a bad yeast infection for the past two months, which one of my doctors diagnosed as Candida. Is it possible that this is the cause of my hair loss? If the Candida is the cause, will my hair grow back once the yeast problem goes away?

ANSWER:

Candida albicans is a common yeast-like fungus that is found in the mouth, digestive tract, vagina, and on the skin of healthy persons. Often a stressful event or condition will reduce the body's immune response capability, and the Candida population will increase dramatically, which can result in a stubborn Candida infection. While it is possible that the stress of the Candida infection is the cause of your hair loss, it is more likely that the same stressful event that triggered the Candida infection two months ago was the cause of your current hair loss. The stressful event could have been be physical, such as having pneumonia or a heart attack, or it could have been emotional such as acute depression, an IRS audit, divorce, or death in the family. A stressful event can cause hair follicles to shift out of the growth phase into the regression phase and then the resting phase, a condition dermatologists call telogen effluvium. It may take three to six months for the growth cycles to normalize again, but the hair should grow back. A visit to a dermatologist will help determine if some other medical condition such as abnormal thyroid hormone levels or iron deficiency anemia is the cause of your hair loss. If a recent stressful event was the cause, the dermatologist may recommend Rogaine to help stabilize the hair follicles over the next three to six months.

QUESTION FROM A 25-YEAR-OLD FEMALE:

I've lost almost eighty percent of my hair from mental stress Can I recover it?

ANSWER:

The answer depends upon the degree and duration of the stress and the hair loss. If a sudden stressful event occurred, and you experienced massive hair shedding a couple of months later, then yes, most if not all the lost hair will likely grow back on its own after the hair follicles go back to their normal growth cycle. Rogaine can help stimulate the regrowth of recently lost hairs. On the other hand, if repeated or continuous stressful events occurred over several years, and the hair loss continued, you may not be able to achieve a full recovery. You should work on learning to be more balanced when faced with stress. Depending upon your situation, a psychiatric professional may be able to assist you, and you may also consider other stress-management techniques such as yoga or meditation. A visit to a dermatologist will help determine if a medical condition may also be contributing to your severe hair loss, and if so medication may be prescribed.

QUESTION FROM A 27-YEAR-OLD FEMALE:

My hair has been shedding for about four years now, and is half the thickness it was in my early twenties. I lose over 100 hairs a day.

I've been to my doctor, had my iron levels and thyroid checked and there is not a single female in my family who had this condition, so it is not hereditary. I've been tested for celiac and many auto immune diseases, all tests have come up negative. Up until a year ago, I was only shedding the longer hairs, but over the past year, I've noticed that even the new, shorter hairs are falling out as much as the longer ones. Many of the new ones are very thin, and seem to have hardly any bulb at the end. Any suggestions?

ANSWER:

It sounds as if you have had the whole list of tests. I would still be concerned about a low serum ferritin. The "normal" range most frequently listed by laboratories is between ten and 230. A report by D. H. Rushton in 2002 correlated the serum ferritin to hair loss. The conclusion was that a level below seventy would make you prone to hair loss. Ask your doctor to order this test. If it is low you can start iron supplements. Another possibility is that you have a diffuse alopecia areata, which may be able to be diagnosed by doing a biopsy and having a hair expert dermatopathologist look at the slides of the sectioned hairs cut horizontally.

QUESTION FROM A 35-YEAR-OLD FEMALE:

Is there any vitamin or herbal product that I can take to stop my hair from shedding?

ANSWER:

No, there are no vitamins or herbal products that have been proven to be effective at reducing reduce hair shedding. All hairs are shed eventually as part of the normal cycle of hair growth, and vitamins and herbal products do not affect the hair growth cycle. If you are experiencing sudden hair shedding, the best treatment for you may be Rogaine, which helps stabilize the hair follicles when they have been stressed and all start losing hairs at the same time. A physical or emotionally stressful event a month or two earlier may now be causing the shedding you are experiencing, a condition dermatologists call telogen effluvium. Rogaine acts as "life support" for the stressed hair follicles, and can prevent continued shedding until the condition stabilizes over a period of months. You should visit a dermatologist for an examination to make sure you are not losing hair because of some medical problem such as a thyroid condition or iron deficiency anemia.

QUESTION FROM A 35-YEAR-OLD FEMALE:

I have some hair loss, but all my hormone levels have been tested and are normal. My doctor has prescribed Ortho Tri-Cyclen birth control pills and says it should help reduce the hair loss. I know some birth control pills actually cause hair loss. What is your advice?

ANSWER:

Hormone levels can fluctuate, and these fluctuations can sometimes have a noticeable effect on the hair follicles. It is true that some birth control pills can cause increased hair loss in some patients, and there are probably a few women who will experience it with Ortho Tri-Cyclen. Ortho Tri-Cyclen is one of the best medications for evening out women's hormone levels and as a result it can help correct thinning hair on the scalp, as well as control hormone-induced acne and excessive facial hair growth. As your doctor said, "it should help,". There are no guarantees in medicine. I recommend that you follow your doctor's advice for nine to twelve months and observe the results. Hair only grows about a half inch per month, and it may take three to four months for some of your resting hair follicles to re-enter the hair growth phase. You may not begin to notice some thickening until six to nine months after you start treatment. Also, you may want to try topical Rogaine in addition to the therapy prescribed by your doctor.

QUESTION FROM A 38-YEAR-OLD FEMALE:

For over a year my hair has been thinning, which was thought to be from surgery. My blood was tested and my iron count was low, so I have been on iron for a year. The hair is still thinning. I also feel cold easily, have dry skin, am tired a lot, have been recently losing weight, but I was gaining, but all the tests show my thyroid is okay. I am using Rogaine with no effect. No one else in my family is losing hair. Why can mine be thinning at thirty-eight, and what can I do?

ANSWER:

Stress from surgery can cause sudden shedding a few months after surgery and can age the hair follicles prematurely. Iron deficiency anemia can also contribute to hair loss and to premature hair follicle aging. It is possible that you have aged your hair follicles so that at age thirty-eight you have the hair you would have had at age fifty-eight. It is also possible that some other illness is contributing to your condition, so I would recommend that you continue to work toward better overall health. Rogaine helps you to keep the hair you have, as well as to help you to grow back recently lost hair a bit thicker and faster. It may take six to nine months before you notice an improvement, so I recommend that you continue the Rogaine treatment.

QUESTION FROM A 40-YEAR-OLD FEMALE:

I had my thyroid hormone levels tested because I was experiencing heavy and prolonged periods. I was placed on medication to correct a hypothyroid condition. Over the past years I have also experienced a great deal of hair thinning, that I think was caused by the thyroid condition. Now that I am on medication to correct my low thyroid hormone level, what are the chances my hair will re-thicken?

ANSWER:

Thyroid hormone imbalances can cause hair loss in some individuals. If your hair loss was caused by your hypothyroid condition and the hair loss was recent, then there is a good chance of getting a lot of it back as a result of medication to treat the thyroid condition. If the hair loss was gradual over a period of several years, the amount of regrowth will likely be small. I recommend that you try Rogaine for at least nine months to see if it can help stop the hair loss and help you grow it back thicker and faster. Hair only grows at a rate of a half inch per month. It may take nine to six months before you notice an improvement, so be patient.

QUESTION FROM A 45-YEAR-OLD FEMALE:

I just had a physical and blood tests, and was diagnosed as having a severely low red blood cell count, but my thyroid was normal. Over the last year I have noticed a large increase in hair loss. Do you think there is a relationship between the anemia and the hair loss, or is this just a reaction to hormonal changes at my age.

Answer:

Anemia is the decreased ability of the red blood cells to provide adequate oxygen supplies to body tissues, including the hair follicles. Anemia may be due to a decreased number of red blood cells, or a decreased amount of various substances in the red blood cells, such as iron, that are necessary for red blood cells to transport oxygen. It is quite possible that your anemia is the primary cause of your hair loss condition, hormone changes could also be playing a role. My advice is to discuss your hair loss symptoms with your physician. Treatment to correct your anemia could very well correct your hair loss condition, it make take six months or longer before you notice an improvement. Ask your doctor for a serum ferritin test and, if indicated, try to get your ferritin level back into the middle of the normal range. You may also try Rogaine to slow the rate of loss until your red blood cell count improves.

Question from a 47-Year-Old Female:

I have hair loss, "male pattern baldness," although neither my mother nor grandmothers had it. I am under a lot of stress right now, and am taking an SSRI antidepressant—Effexor. All of my blood work has come back "normal." Doctor started me on spirolactone (100 mg/day) and OrthoCylen birth control pills for the hormone effect. So far, after one month I don't see any results. I have been on the Atkins Diet this past month, too, and just today I read that some people on the diet lose hair and that even Dr. Atkins himself warns of this on his website. I have been taking a daily vitamin called Centrum, plus a "hair vitamin" which tastes terrible, and 5000 mcg of saw palmetto. I also take one B complex a day. I have here a list of other supplements I feel I should buy that I have read about—for example biotin, flax seed oil, and even prenatal vitamins—but have not gotten any more supplements as the ones I have don't seem to be helping. My hair just keeps getting thinner. I don't know if it is from stress or what. I started to lose my hair in my twenties, but it has only now become visible because my hair was so very thick when I was younger. But now I have the actual male pattern baldness and you can see the bald spots in certain areas. Do you know of anything I can do to nourish my hair? Is there something I can do to keep it from falling out or even growing back?

Answer:

There are many possible causes for your hair loss: 1) inherited baldness from either side of your family, 2) chronic stress, 3) low serum ferritin, 4) antidepressants, 5) hormonal imbalance. It looks as if your doctor has you on the right medications to prevent more loss due to inherited androgenic alopecia and hormonal problems. You did not mention the degree of hair loss your father had. In any case, you can have inherited balding genes from both sides and end up having the thinnest head of hair in the family. I would suggest you use Rogaine to help the loss due to stress. I will take four to six months to see new hair growth due to these medical treatments. Hair loss due to dieting would come under the heading of loss due to stress and is usually the starvation dieting where you would lose thirty or more pounds a month. If that is not the case I would not think Atkins diet is the cause.

Since your hair loss began before you began taking your SSRI antidepressant it may not be the cause. Ask your doctor about your serum ferritin level. It should be above sixty even though most laboratories list twenty to 150 as normal. If you are low the treatment with ferrous sulfate 325 milligrams a day may help. I do not think the other supplements and hair vitamins will be of any value.

Question from a 48-Year-Old Female:

About fourteen years ago as a result of a severe viral illness with very high fever, night sweats, vomiting, and incessant coughing, my hair started to fall out. I assumed it was due to acute telogen effluvium and that the situation would right itself in due course. This is not so. I am not bald because new hairs grow immediately after an old one is shed, but the anagen phase seems to be very short. Some of the shed hairs are new—less than one centimeter long. Is there anything that can be done?

ANSWER:

It certainly sounds as if you had severe telogen effluvium. When the anagen (growth) phase becomes short, it is usually a sign of androgenetic alopecia, inherited pattern hair loss. It is possible that your telogen effluvium episode accelerated the date when some of your hair follicles would shorten their growth phase. These hairs follicles will eventually stop producing hairs altogether. I recommend that you try Rogaine to help prolong the anagen phase of the affected hairs, which will then allow the hairs they produce to grow longer. Apply it across the front, and very thinly. Leave the sides along, as the medication will find its way there.

QUESTION FROM A 54-YEAR-OLD FEMALE:

I had a great deal of stress over the past three months and then I noticed that my hair was all over the desk at work, my chair, and at home. I had some tests done and my thyroid is a little on the low side but the doctor decided to leave it alone. I also had two other episodes of alopecia areata (patchy hair loss) when taking care of my ill mother. My dermatologist at the time said that I might have other episodes of this, but that I should just get the treatments and that I would recover the hair. I have had the shots recently, and the hair seems to have stopped falling out in massive amounts. I also had a biopsy done and it came back as "androgenetic alopecia" which I tend to disagree with, since I have always had hair regrowth with the shots. I have been doing a lot of research and have been desperate for the last two weeks. What do you think?

ANSWER:

It sounds as if you had a classic case of telogen effluvium. The timing of the loss and subsequent thinning is consistent with that diagnosis. The diagnosis of androgenetic alopecia, inherited pattern hair loss, is also quite possible. Usually four to five months after an incident of telogen effluvium or alopecia areata, the hair follicles begin to grow new hairs again, however each hair follicle is programmed to have only so many "lives" and repeated stressful events that cause pre-mature shedding can use up some of these "lives" and age the hair follicles. The result can be an inherited condition such as androgenetic alopecia showing up early, and causing your hair to appear as it would have ten or twenty years from now. The best therapy combination would be to learn to respond better to stress and use Rogaine to help stabilize and stimulate the hair follicles.

QUESTION FROM A 55-YEAR-OLD FEMALE:

I am going in for chemotherapy and my doctor mentioned there is a new medicine that could protect my hair. What can you tell me about this?

ANSWER:

A group of dermatologists discussed the issue of a drug being developed by the pharmaceutical company Glaxo Wellcome (now GlaxoSmithKline) that may in the future help cancer patients undergoing chemotherapy suffer less hair loss.

The medication has been applied on rats as a topical cream several hours before chemotherapy to effectively protect hairs from falling out after chemotherapy treatment. According to the discussion group participants, the research has been reported on BBC News Online, PBS McNeil Lehrer Report, and in the journal *Science*. According to the discussion group participants, cancer patients who responded to a survey by Glaxo Wellcome ranked hair loss as second only to nausea and vomiting as the most unpleasant side effect of their chemotherapy treatment. A quote attributed to Professor Gordon McVie, Director General of the Cancer Research Campaign in the United Kingdom, included: "Without a doubt (chemotherapy induced hair loss) contributes to a deteriorating self-image, and many patients do not believe that their hair will ever grow back even if they are told it is a temporary phenomenon."

MY COMMENT:

This medication presents a trade off of benefit versus risk. Chemotherapy works by targeting rapidly dividing cells typical of cancerous growth, but also affects other fast-growing cells such as those that produce the hair shaft inside the hair follicles. It appears the mechanism of action of the anti-hair loss drug is to temporarily slow or stop cell division in the hair follicles, which protects them from absorbing the chemotherapy medication. This would likely also protect cancerous cells from the chemotherapy medication, if they were in or around the hair follicles. If the chemotherapy is intended only to shrink or eliminate a cancerous tumor located away from the scalp, and the tumor is the type that does not present a significant risk of metastases to the skin, then the benefits may outweigh the risks. But there is evidence to suggest that many basal cell carcinomas, the most common type of human tumor, originate in the hair follicles. If there were a risk that the cancer being treated originated in the skin or could spread to the skin and hair follicles of the scalp, then it would be best for the chemotherapy medication to be allowed to fully affect those cells as well, in order to protect the patient from the possibility of metastatic cancer cells in the hair follicles.

QUESTION FROM A 58-YEAR-OLD FEMALE:

I'm losing my hair fast! I've been worrying about it a lot. Maybe I need hormone pills. Is there anything I can do to help this problem?

ANSWER:

Yes, if low hormone levels are the cause of your hair loss, there are effective treatments available. By age fifty-eight many women begin to experience hair thinning due to changes in estrogen hormone levels. Women can inherit a tendency for hair loss just as men do, and around age thirty these women will have increased blood levels of the hormone DHT telling their hair follicles to stop growing new hairs, just as would be the case in men who inherited male pattern baldness. Young women high levels of estrogen hormones interfere with the DHT message, and "protect" the susceptible hair follicles. But later in life, as estrogen levels decline, the DHT message eventually gets through to the susceptible follicles, and thinning hair is the result.

Often estrogen supplements, or oral contraceptives such as Ortho Tri-Cyclen that have a significant effect on estrogen hormone levels, can stop the hair thinning. Elevating estrogen levels to control hair loss is a treatment method that is applicable only to women, as it would have undesirable side effects on men. Also, if your blood pressure is normal or a bit high, your doctor may prescribe spironolactone, a medication that is used to lower blood pressure, but will also help to block the hormones telling the hair follicles to stop growing. You should consult with a dermatologist, as well as your primary care physician, to be sure that hormone levels are the only cause of your hair loss.

QUESTION FROM A 58-YEAR-OLD FEMALE:

Why is it that some of my hair is brown, while most of it is gray? How is it determined which hair grays?

ANSWER:

Hair color, like eye color, is genetically determined. Many people naturally experience hair color changes over their lifetime. Infants with light colored hair sometimes develop darker colored hair within a year or two, and vice versa. Certain hair follicles are genetically programmed to begin growing gray hairs after a certain number of growth cycles. In men the hair follicles at the temples, sideburns, beard, and mustache will often become gray before the hair at the back of the head. In women the pattern of gray hair is usually more generalized. There have been some cases noted where trauma from an injury or emotional shock has accelerated the graying process, but this is rare. Environmental factors such as sunlight, chlorine in swimming pools, and hair dyes can affect the appearance of hair color, without affecting the color of the hair that the hair follicles are producing.

Some stem cells that generate the cells which make pigment—producing blondes, brunettes and redheads—die off with age. Cell survival in general is influenced by an "anti-death" gene known as Bcl2. It could be that people who gray prematurely have a genetic program that knocks out Bcl2

QUESTION FROM A 65-YEAR-OLD FEMALE:

Last year I underwent two lumpectomies for breast cancer. I had six months of chemotherapy, followed by six weeks of radiation treatment, and lost all of my hair. My hair started growing back within a few months and had a loose curl and was very manageable. But six months later I have noticed fallout at the roots, not breakage, in my brush and comb. My hair now also appears to be oily, a condition I never had before. I am very distressed by this situation. Is this condition cancer-related?

ANSWER:

I doubt that your falling hair and increased oiliness is due to an ongoing cancer. It is more likely that it is due to accelerated aging of the hair follicles as a result of your cancer treatment, with the result that you now have the hair at age sixty-five that you would have had at age eighty-five. Your oily hair condition may also be due to stress or changes in your diet or perhaps from drug interactions. I recommend that you schedule an appointment with a dermatologist to have your scalp examined, and be sure to bring along a complete list of all medications you are currently taking.

QUESTION ON BEHALF OF A 10-YEAR-OLD MALE:

My grandson, who is ten years old, was burned in a house fire at the age of three months. He is bald on the top and partially on one side from this, and his skin is also very thin on top of his head because several layers of skin were burned off. He is made fun of every day. Would he be a good candidate for hair restoration surgery?

ANSWER:

I recently treated a thirteen-year-old girl with a similar problem. I would need to see photos of the child's scalp showing the extent of the damaged area to best evaluate what I think could be done. I would expect that he could benefit from the removal of some scar tissue and then receive a modest amount of hair transplantation. Keep in mind that he would be his own donor, and hair transplantation surgery only redistributes the patient's own hair follicles to give the appearance of a fuller head of hair.

The age at which surgery is performed depends upon how motivated the child would be to sit through several procedures spaced a few months apart, with each lasting several hours. We use local anesthesia to numb the scalp, along with a tranquilizer tablet, a sleeping pill, and a pain pill, but no general anesthesia, meaning the patient is very relaxed but awake during the procedure. While I understand how troubling his condition can be to you, and the emotional challenge the child faces from teasing by classmates at school, I usually tell parents to wait until the child asks to have the scar tissue removed in his or her early teenage years.

QUESTION FROM AN 18-YEAR-OLD MALE:

I am having hair loss. My father is almost bald, and he is fifty years old. I've started doing Sirsasana (headstand) to increase blood flow to the scalp. I have also started putting my own morning urine on my scalp because I read that it will reduce hair loss, but no regrowth. I heard about Fabao and Kevis. Is it good? Does it work?

ANSWER:

Of the various treatments you have described, none of them sounds worthwhile to me. You should see a dermatologist, a doctor who specializes in treating conditions affecting the skin, hair and nails, and if it is determined that genetics is the likely cause of your hair loss, you should get a prescription for Propecia, which is the best way to slow and stop inherited hair loss. Rogaine may also help the hair you have grow a little better, longer and thicker.

QUESTION FROM A 20-YEAR-OLD MALE:

How can I stop or slow down the thinning process in the front of my hair, and how can I stop the receding hairline? I am very scared about losing my hair! Please help, and thanks.

ANSWER:

An examination by a dermatologist will determine if your hair loss is caused by inherited male pattern baldness. If this is the cause of your hair loss, Propecia would be the most effective therapy for slowing, stopping, and even reversing the thinning you are experiencing. Propecia is most effective when started at an early age.

QUESTION FROM A 20-YEAR-OLD MALE:

My hair is very thin. It is not growing properly. I am very upset to face this problem. I like growing long thick hair. Sir, my hair is very thin. All my friends are laughing at me for facing this problem at this age. Please kindly HELP me out of this problem. Please mention some remedies to grow thick long hair. Please tell me what I should use to grow THICK, long hair. Can I use Hair Formula 37 to get thick long hair?

ANSWER:

You need to see a dermatologist to determine if this is an inherited condition, or some other type of medical condition. Depending upon the cause of the hair loss, a dermatologist may be able to prescribe a medication such as Propecia to slow your loss, and possibly help your hair grow back.

QUESTION FROM A 23-YEAR-OLD MALE:

I'm developing male pattern baldness i.e. a receding hairline, and daily I consider which surgery would suit me best. I'm considering laser surgery at a clinic.

ANSWER:

Before considering any form of surgery, see a dermatologist who will sit down with you and explain the role Propecia can play in slowing your hair loss condition. Propecia may help you get the hair back that you recently lost, and may be able to help stop future hair loss. Do not go to a laser clinic first. Lasers are expensive pieces of equipment, and have to be used for procedures to be paid for. You may end up with scars from laser surgery that are more difficult to hide than your thin hair spots.

QUESTION FROM A 24-YEAR-OLD MALE:

If I get transplants, will my hair loss be in the loss condition it is now when I am forty-eight? Or is hair loss reversible, or is there a stopping to it advancing?

ANSWER:

Without medical treatment, hair loss is a progressive condition, meaning that it will continue as you age. For some people the rate of loss is slow, and for others it is quite rapid. Hair transplantation is not usually done on patients at age twenty-four because it is very difficult to predict the degree and rate of future loss at the early stages of pattern hair loss. Also, there are now medical treatments such as Propecia, which can be prescribed by a dermatologist, and can be very effective at stopping hair loss at an early age. If you still have some hair loss, such as a receding hairline, after being on Propecia for several years, a hair restoration surgeon will be able to evaluate your hair loss condition, and then you may consider transplants if desired.

The following three questions all have the same answer:

QUESTION FROM A 23-YEAR-OLD MALE:

What specifically causes facial hair? I personally am not going bald. However, I have a problem producing a full mustache and beard. Is there a vitamin or medication that can help me with this?

QUESTION FROM A 25-YEAR-OLD MALE:

I still haven't got proper growth of hair on my body. I have scant mustache and very little beard without any whiskers. I don't have much hair on my arms and legs, though I have hair on my groin area. I feel very shy at times. I have checked up my hormone levels and they are normal. I don't have any other problems with anything, e.g. sexual matters. Is there any lotion, medication, or treatment with which I could grow dark mustache and beard? I have become quite introverted due to this thing. Please show me a way to get rid of this.

QUESTION FROM A 27-YEAR-OLD MALE:

From the age of eighteen, I started to lose hairs, and I tried many medicines but all in vain. My father and his brothers are all bald but my two elder brothers and one younger brother do not have any problems with hairs. Why is it that I lost all my hairs?

ANSWER:

Pattern baldness is inherited in much the same way as height is inherited. You may be the tallest or the shortest person in your family, depending upon the combination of genes you get from your father and your mother, and your brothers may have inherited slightly different genes. You may have inherited balding genes from your mother as well as your father, and she may not show any hair thinning because she is female and has low levels of the hormone that tells the hair to fall out. Your brothers may have inherited slightly different genes that affect hair loss. If your family does not show baldness on both sides, you should see a dermatologist to determine if your hair loss could be caused by some illness.

Question from a 28-Year-Old Male:

I am losing my hair. I have noticed my bathroom is full of hair after I take a shower. I don't know what to do. I am scared to death. I am afraid to look in the mirror. I have always had very, very thick hair. And in only a few weeks I can see my head through my hair. I am afraid to go to doctors because I don't want to use any chemical creams or pills to kill my hair. I have never used shampoo in my life. I have started washing my hair with egg yolk from organic eggs. Please help!

Answer:

Despite your reluctance to see a doctor, you should see a dermatologist so you can be examined for conditions that may be the cause of your hair loss. A dermatologist will examine your scalp and hair, and ask the appropriate questions to determine if further tests are needed. The sudden shedding you are experiencing may be just a temporary condition, and could have been caused by a stressful event such as a bad cold or emotional stress six or more weeks ago, and is only now causing your hair loss. But see a dermatologist to be sure. The therapy suggested to you by any dermatologist is not going to kill your hair, and it may help save it.

Question from a 29-Year-Old Male:

I am noticing a rapid increase in the amount of hair I'm losing. I have no bald spots yet, but my hairline is receding and the hair at the top and back of my head is becoming much thinner. I am not interested in hair transplants, but would consider either Propecia or Rogaine. Which product would you recommend?

Answer:

There is no question about it; Propecia is the medication for you. It is the only drug that has been clinically tested in carefully controlled studies and has been proven to actually prevent the hair follicles from getting the message to grow old and stop growing hairs. Rogaine, another drug, seems to tell the hair follicles to keep growing hair, even though they are still getting the message to die. If you were to use Rogaine for ten years, and then stop using it, you would have a heavy shedding of hairs within a few months. These hairs would have been lost if not for the Rogaine keeping them alive. But Propecia seems to work by preventing the message from getting to the hair follicles in the first place. If you were to stop using Propecia tablets after ten years, your hair loss would again begin gradually, but your hair follicles would be ten years "younger" as a result of the Propecia treatment.

QUESTION FROM A 30-YEAR-OLD MALE:

When I look at before/after pictures of people who have transplants, it seems like they never show the crown area in the "after" pics. I'm always wondering—are they trying to hide something? My thinnest area is the crown and it really bothers me. Realistically how dense could I expect the hair on my crown to be if I had transplants?

ANSWER:

With a few sessions of follicular unit micrografting transplants, your crown could approach the same density as the surrounding area; however, transplantation to the crown is not often promoted for three good reasons:

First, most hair loss patients are concerned about how they look from the front, which is how they see themselves in a mirror, as well as how others see them head-on. I know from decades of experience that there are many men who are balding both at the hairline as well as at the crown, and it is true that some of these men express more concern about their "bald spot" at the crown, than their receding hairlines. But the vast majority of balding men are more concerned with how they look from the front, than the back. This does not mean that your concern is not real, and there are several options for treating hair loss at the crown, including transplants.

Second, all hair transplantation techniques involve moving a limited supply of donor hairs from the back and sides of the head, to other locations such as to the hairline and crown, where they will have a greater visual impact, and create a look of a fuller head of hair. Most men with hair loss begin to first lose hair at their hairlines, and later begin to have thin hair on top, and eventually may have baldness on their crown. However, some men begin to lose hair first at the crown, and then later may experience hair loss at the hairline. Promoting hair transplantation to the crown area is a sure way to bring in more patients who will have unrealistic expectations of what the doctor can do to correct their hair loss. If the limited supply of donor hair is used up densely filling the crown area, there may be no way to address a receding hairline years later as the hair loss progresses. While some hair restoration surgeons think all patients should be told simply to "leave the back alone," I evaluate each patient on a case by case basis and take into consideration their age, current and projected hair loss, and whether the patient will use medication to reduce future hair loss. Generally the front area gets the most grafts, while the top of the head receives a smaller proportion of transplants.

Medication is the third reason for little promotion of transplantation to the crown area. Both Rogaine and Propecia, the only medications that have been proven in clinical trials to be effective at reducing hair loss, are most effective on the crown. If you review the literature describing the effectiveness of these two medications, you will see that most of the examples involve the crown area. Of the two, Propecia is most effective for stopping hair loss, and in many cases restores hair growth to follicles that recently stopped growing new hairs. Propecia can reduce the need for transplantation to the crown area. I consider a patient with some thinning at the crown who takes Propecia, to be a better candidate for transplantation to the crown area than if they did not take the medication.

Question from a 30-Year-Old Male:

If I get transplants how real will they look? Will I be able to grow my hair as long as I want? Will I have to keep going back to a clinic for check-ups or "re-adjustment" of my transplants? If I choose to keep shaving my head will people be able to tell that I had a transplant?

ANSWER:

These are excellent questions. Transplanted hair using the follicular micrograft technique looks very natural because the hairs grow from the scalp in much the same way that they do naturally. The transplanted hair follicles will be removed in the form of a strip of tissue from the scalp at the back of your head, which will be separated into follicular unit micrografts containing one to three hairs, and the individual grafts will be placed into tiny incisions on the front and top of your scalp. The transplanted hair follicles will continue to grow new hairs in the locations they are moved to. On the top and front of the scalp, the transplanted follicles will grow hair just as long as they would have at the original location on the back of the scalp. Hair grows about a half inch per month, so it may take two years to grow hair a foot long, but if that's what you want, you can do it.

About a week after a transplant procedure, you would return to the surgeon's office for an examination to make sure that the transplanted follicles are growing properly, and that there are no complications, and to have sutures at the donor area at the back of your scalp removed. After that, there is no real need for additional check-ups, and with a skilled and artistically capable surgeon, no need for "readjustments." Each follicular unit micrograft procedure is designed to stand alone, and to look natural for the rest of your life, even if you continue to lose hair and never have any more work done. Depending upon the degree of hair loss you have currently, one procedure may be adequate; many patients choose to have additional procedures done to achieve increased hair density at the hairline and on top.

If you were to shave your head completely some time after a follicular micrograft procedure, the transplant would be detectable. The donor area would appear as a single fine line scar running across the back of your scalp. This scar may not be especially noticeable because it follows the natural skin folds that occur when you tilt your head back, and I use two sets of sutures to close the donor site to create the thinnest possible scar. One set of sutures are placed below the surface of the skin to relieve tension on the wound and are made with dissolving thread, and the second set of sutures close the donor site opening at the surface with removable stitches. Also, when a second or third procedure is performed, the existing scar is removed, so there would never be more than a single fine line at the donor site.

The tiny incisions on the front and top of the scalp made for each micrograft may or may not be visible if you were to shave your head completely. The individual incisions are very small, and are made with a very fine surgical blade designed for eye surgery. The degree of visible scarring at the recipient sites is largely dependant upon your skin type, and your tendency to scar. People of African, Asian, and Native American descent typically have more pronounced scarring than do people of European heritage. I had a patient of European descent who had over 300 micrografts placed to enhance his mustache, and when his job situation required him to shave off his mustache, he had no visible scars. But not every transplant patient will be so fortunate.

QUESTION FROM A 32-YEAR-OLD MALE:

I have a mustache and a goatee, and they are quite thick, I guess. But the hairs on the sides of my face are not that thick. Moreover, on one side of my face, there is hardly any hair for stubble for a side burn. What can be done to correct this? Is there something genetically wrong with me? Some people mistake me for a woman on the phone, so I guess there is something wrong with my voice. I've tried applying Rogaine on my face, but I don't think it helped much. I know this is probably silly and making me seem vain, but being able to grow a beard is as important to me as a woman being able to give birth to a baby. I feel insufficient as a man because of this. Can you please help me?

ANSWER:

Facial hair, as well as all other hair distribution on the body, is determined by your genetics. There are no vitamins or medications that are safe and effective at stimulating facial hair growth.

Some men have had hair transplants to enhance a mustache or beard. The problem is, we cannot be sure that if the patient shaves there will be no marks or scars showing where the transplanted hairs are growing. I had one patient, a twenty-five-year-old clerk, who came to me because he wanted a full mustache. We did 300 grafts and he was tickled pink with the result. Later, he joined a more conservative firm that required a clean-shaven look. Fortunately, in his case, the transplants were not obvious when he shaved his mustache, but this is not always so.

QUESTION FROM A 33-YEAR-OLD MALE:

This is going to sound like a really weird question, but for about five years now I have been noticing that I seem to be losing a lot of hair (sink, shower, brush) but still have a full head of hair and no thinning spots. Am I just being paranoid because I'm at that age? Is there a reason I'm losing so much hair but it doesn't ever show?

ANSWER:

Everyone is born with about 100,000 hairs on his or her head, and about half of them can be lost before the hair begins to looks thin. Each hair is shed eventually, and after a resting period, a new hair begins to grow from the same hair follicle where the old hair was shed. An average of fifty to 100 hairs are shed every day, and approximately the same number of new hairs start growing each day. Since you still have a full head of hair with no thinning spots, you are most likely experiencing normal shedding.

QUESTION FROM A 33-YEAR-OLD MALE:

I've been losing a tremendous amount of hair every day but show no signs of thinning anywhere. I went to see my Dermatologist, and he told me I have "normal hair density" and that I am probably one of the few people with very short shedding cycle" and that I would probably never be able to grow long hair (which I haven't). Could you please tell me what all this means?

ANSWER:

We all start out with about 100,000 active hair follicles. On average about fifty to 100 hairs are shed every day, and fifty to 100 new hairs begin growing each day as well. Typically a new hair grows about a half inch a month for about five years, which would allow a hair to grow about thirty inches long if it was not cut during that time. After an average of five years, the hair follicle goes into regression and resting phases for a few months, during which the hair is usually shed.

After a few more months, a new hair again begins to grow from the same hair follicle, and the growth cycle starts over. Typically about ninety percent of the hair follicles are growing hair, while the other ten percent are shedding or resting. Some people have a genetic program for a shorter average growing cycle, perhaps only two or three years, while others have longer average growing cycles. A shorter average growing cycle would result in hairs being shed before they could grow as long as thirty inches. It would also result in greater hair shedding, as a higher percentage of the 100,000 hair follicles would be in the shedding phase, when compared to a person with a longer growth cycle. The person with the shorter growing cycle would also have a higher percentage of new hairs starting to grow each day, but this would be a lot less noticeable than seeing the shed hairs in the sink and shower drain.

Question from a 39-Year-Old Male:

My mom's dad had a head full of hair. My dad's dad went bald, and my dad is bald himself. Do I have the chance of going bald? I used to have really thick hair but it seems to be thinning. I do use hair styling products. What should I use? What can I do to prevent hair loss?

Answer:

The genetic predisposition to have hair loss can be passed on by either or both parents. If your father is bald and his father also became bald, then you have a good chance of also suffering pattern baldness. Hair styling products are cosmetic, meaning they only affect appearance and will have no effect on your hair loss. The best way to address your hair loss is to see a dermatologist, and if an exam determines that your thinning hair is due to genetics, a prescription for Propecia can help to stop and possibly reverse the hair loss you are experiencing.

Question from a 39-Year-Old Male:

I heard that men lose hair because hair follicles either become dead or dormant. My question is what determines whether they become dead or just dormant?

Answer:

Over time, a naturally-occurring hormone in the blood of both men and women called dihydrotestosterone, usually abbreviated DHT, signals certain hair follicles that have been genetically programmed for hair loss to slowly stop producing new hairs. So the answer to your question is that a combination of DHT and genetics and time all determine which hair follicles stop growing hairs. DHT in the blood gets to all the hair follicles on the body. Only the ones that are genetically programmed to be sensitive to the DHT message stop growing hairs. In men with pattern hair loss, these follicles are usually located at the hairline and on the top of the head. In women, the DHT-sensitive hair follicles are distributed more generally over the top of the head.

Initially, most hair follicles affected by DHT seem to be "dormant," and if the DHT message is quickly blocked by medication such as Propecia, or a competing message to grow occurs, such as with the medication Rogaine, some of the dormant follicles will awaken and begin to grow new hairs again. However, if the DHT message is allowed to continue, over time the "dormant" follicles cannot be awakened and may be considered "dead." The exact biochemical changes that occur when a hair follicle goes from being productive, to dormant, to unproductive, are not completely understood. But we do know that medical treatment at the early stages of hair loss is more effective than treatment at later stages.

Question from a 41-Year-Old Male:

I have three children and a wife, and have what I consider to be a lot of premature wrinkling spots below my lower lip off to the sides. This coincides with areas where I have bald spots in my beard area. I grew a goatee beard, except that it did not look good due to these bald spots. I was wondering if you have ever done hair transplants on facial areas such as this. Is there scarring? Is this a nutty idea?

Answer:

Certainly some people consider facial hair transplants to be a nutty idea, however they have been performed in Japan since the

1930s, and on occasion in this country since that time to correct injuries from burns and accidents. I receive a surprising number of inquiries about enhancing facial hair growth from men in their twenties and thirties who believe that if only they had a thicker mustache or beard, their lives would be different. I do not advise transplants for these young men.

Facial hair transplants involve the same theory of donor dominance that scalp hair transplants are based upon. Donor hair follicles are taken from the back of the head, and moved in this instance to the face, rather than to the scalp. The transplanted hair follicles will continue to grow hairs at the new location, based upon their genetic program. I perform mustache and beard enhancing facial hair transplants on occasion for mature men who have a good understanding of the benefits and risks of such a procedure. The procedure involves carefully placing hundreds of single-hair grafts between existing hair follicles in the mustache or beard area. The benefits, of course, are thicker facial hair. The risks include using up some of the limited supply of donor hairs, as well as the risk of small but visible scars at the recipient area. Also, the transplanted hairs may have a somewhat different texture than the existing facial hair, and may need to be trimmed more frequently. On my web site you can view photos of a man who received transplants to his mustache area, and was quite satisfied with the results. Some time after the transplant procedure, he got a job at a law firm that required a clean-shaven appearance of all employees, and he shaved off his enhanced mustache. He was fortunate in that his skin did not show visible scars from the tiny incisions that were made for the facial hair grafts. Others may have more visible scarring, should they choose to shave off their enhanced facial hair.

QUESTION FROM A 48-YEAR-OLD MALE:

I am using both Proscar 5mg/day (tablets) and minoxidil (lotion) double strength twice a day. It seems that I am growing new hair with some gain in the back and somewhat less in the front. Has this combination been proven to be effective? Is one better than the other? Any dosage recommendations or other advice?

ANSWER:

Proscar is the brand name for the drug finasteride when it is prescribed as a pill for treating enlarged prostate glands. The same drug finasteride, in a lower dosage, is FDA approved in tablet form for treating hair loss under the brand name Propecia. Since you are taking Proscar, I would assume it was prescribed to treat a prostate gland condition, and you are enjoying the desirable side effect of reduced hair loss.

Minoxidil is the active ingredient drug in Rogaine, which in lotion form was originally available by prescription only, and is now FDA approved as an "over-the-counter" medicine for treating hair loss. Minoxidil lotion is not absorbed well into the skin, and excessive application can cause skin irritation. For treating hair loss, the combination of oral finasteride and topical minoxidil is more effective than either one used alone, and this combination has been used since 1993. A study of the effectiveness of the drug combination was published in a dermatology journal a year or two later. Simply put, finasteride works by stopping most of the DHT hormone message telling the hair follicles to stop growing. Minoxidil works by telling the follicles to keep growing hairs, even when they get the DHT hormone message. My advice would be to continue your present treatment. Between the two medications, it is the finasteride in your Proscar tablets which will help you most in the long run.

The following two questions have the same answer.

QUESTION FROM A 59-YEAR-OLD MALE:

Although I use a dandruff shampoo, I still have a flaky itchy scalp. What can I do?

QUESTION FROM A 41-YEAR-OLD MALE:

I am troubled by dandruff. Although I wash my hair frequently (four to five times a week), my dandruff tends to reoccur. Why does this happen? Is there a way to permanently cure dandruff? I've heard that some dandruff shampoos actually make dandruff worse in the long run. What causes dandruff? What can I do?

ANSWER:

Dandruff is a common condition, and surprisingly the cause is not well understood. First, let me state that dandruff does not cause hair loss, nor is it a symptom of hair loss. Also, there is no permanent cure for dandruff, but it can be controlled fairly easily. Dandruff is a condition characterized by excessive scaling and skin flake shedding on the scalp. Dandruff is sometimes accompanied by an itching sensation, and sometimes by excessive oiliness, but without visible redness or inflammation. Dermatologists call excessive oiliness on the skin seborrhea. Excessive scaling and skin flaking accompanied by visible redness and inflammation, usually occurring in areas where the skin is oily, is called seborrheic dermatitis. Flaking on the scalp, without redness, is dandruff.

Dead skin cells on the surface of scalp, just like skin cells on the surface everywhere else on the body, are eventually shed as new skin cells grow out from the underlying layers of skin. Normally a new skin cell grows from the innermost layer of skin, and as older skin cells are shed in an orderly manner, after about a month the new skin cell reaches the surface layers and eventually dies and is shed itself. And normally, the dead skin cells fall off a few layers at a time, in tiny clusters that are microscopic and not noticed.

With dandruff, there is a combination of an uneven rate of skin cell growth and abnormally sticky sebum (hair oil) that result in comparatively large flakes of skin twenty to forty layers thick being shed. These relatively large chunks of dead skin cells are visible as dandruff flakes.

Although the exact cause of dandruff is not completely understood, the condition is associated with an increase in the population of certain microorganisms that naturally occur on the scalp, including Pityrosporum ovale, a yeast-like fungus that lives in the oil glands and hair follicles on the scalp. The cause of the increase in the population of Pityrosporum ovale is not well understood, and dandruff conditions often change over time for an individual, even without treatment. Dermatologists have a range of prescription treatments for dandruff, including medications that control itching, reduce oiliness, slow the rate of skin cell growth, and kill the microorganisms associated with excessive scalp flaking.

The most effective non-prescription dandruff treatments are shampoos with ingredients that reduce the population of these microorganisms. After rinsing off the anti-dandruff shampoos, the active ingredients remain on the surface of the scalp. Furthermore, alternating each day between shampoos with different active ingredients has been shown to be more effective at controlling dandruff than using a single anti-dandruff shampoo product every day.

Before scheduling an appointment with a dermatologist to control your dandruff, try alternating between Nizoral one percent shampoo, containing ketoconazole and now available at drugstores without a prescription, and either a shampoo containing zinc pyrithione such as regular Head & Shoulders, or a shampoo containing selenium sulfide, such as Selsun Blue shampoo. Or try alternating among all three. If, after a few weeks, your dandruff condition does not seem to be improving, then consult with a dermatologist.

QUESTION FROM 42-YEAR-OLD MALE:

I am a management consultant, in the hospital field, with considerable coursework in biology and chemistry. I also sold pharmaceuticals, and I have read extensively in all the sciences. I receive a "Longevity Journal" which this month is touting and selling "Testone Cream" and "Teston 6" capsules. These products contain DHEA and "andro" plus "pregnenolone." I take high blood pressure pills, which depress testosterone, and I do have the genetic trait for male pattern baldness. I am not overly concerned about this, but if I could spend two or three bucks a day to correct my lack of vigor, and correct my increasing baldness, I would do it. But there is just so damn much hype and hucksterism going on that it seems impossible to make sound decisions. I'll be damned if I can evaluate claims outside of the field of formal medicine. Would you share your thoughts on this?

ANSWER:

Worthless products and treatments alleged to cause permanent weight loss, improve sexual vigor, extend the lifespan, cure cancer or AIDS, and of course stop hair loss, cost consumers around the world billions of dollars each year. It is an extremely profitable business for the sellers, and there is very little regulatory control over performance claims.

These "miracle products" inevitably target our fears, hopes, and vanity. Their claims are supported by stories and testimonials, rather than reproducible scientific studies, although some sellers of these products fraudulently claim to have such studies as well. The products may have been "used for years in Europe," or Asia, or somewhere else, and are only now available for purchase in this country. They often explain their effectiveness by inventing a somewhat plausible "cause" for the condition to be treated, and then explain that their product "cures" that particular problem. Effectiveness claims of seventy percent, eighty percent, ninety percent, and more are thrown out with reckless abandon.

The products will invariably list "ingredients" with scientific-sounding names, often similar to medications that are related to treating the condition. They will claim the product is "all natural," "herbal," and "has no side effects." And there will be an offer for a money-back guarantee, if the product for some reason does not work.

It is amazing what even well-educated people will buy. We all hope for a miracle cure, a quick and easy solution to our problems. While you personally may laugh at an advertisement for a product making outlandish promises to erase cellulite or enlarge breasts, you may choose to purchase products with similar claims that are guaranteed to increase your energy level or reverse your hair loss. After all, its only "two or three bucks a day." I have to confess that I myself have a collection of half-a-dozen or so different abdominal exercise devices whose promises of miracle results seemed to make sense at the end of their 2:00 A.M. cable TV infomercials.

The United States Food and Drug Administration (U.S. FDA) is charged with regulating foods, drugs, and cosmetics. But in 1994 the Dietary Supplement Health and Education Act (DSHEA) was passed with massive lobbying by the health-food industry, and this act greatly weakened the ability of the FDA to protect consumers from unsubstantiated claims made by supplement sellers.

In addition, the Federal Trade Commission (FTC) and the United States Postal Service (USPS) have laws intended to regulate truth in advertising and interstate commerce; these laws are rarely enforced, and even when they are enforced, the penalties are small in comparison to the profits generated by the sales of bogus products.

A little common sense will tell you that if a particular product really did have the ability to safely and effectively treat any of these conditions, it would be worth hundreds of millions of dollars or more, and would be marketed in a reputable manner, not on late night TV infomercials, or talk-radio commercials, or by multi-level marketing schemes, or advertisements disguised as "newsletters" or scientific "journals."

The particular "journal" you mention, the *Journal of Longevity,* is published by Almon Glenn Braswell. According to Stephen Barrett, MD, who operates the Quackwatch web site (www.quackwatch.com), Braswell has probably sold more dietary supplements by mail over the past twenty years than any similar marketer in U.S. history. In 1983, Braswell settled a federal lawsuit for $610,000, in which the FTC charged that his company did not have adequate scientific evidence that their hair loss products worked, including a product called "Bio-Genesis," and that they had not paid refunds as promised to their customers (See "FTC News Notes" October 4, 1983).

In 1984 a USPS official summarized at a congressional hearing that 138 false representation complaints were filed against fifty different medical-cosmetic products marketed by Braswell, Inc. One case revealed that Braswell received over $2,000,000 in one six-month period for a worthless baldness cure. Mr. Braswell pled guilty to mail fraud charges involving faking before and after advertising photographs, and was sentenced to five years probation. He was also sentenced to a three-year prison term for federal income tax evasion (See "Quackery: A $10 Billion Scandal" Washington DC: U.S. Government Printing Office, 1984, pages 137-138).

BIO-GENESIS CONTINUES TO BE SOLD TODAY

In July 2000, an article sympathetic to "alternative medicine" attributed to Florida Governor Jeb Bush, appeared in the *Journal of Longevity.* Investigators from *Newsweek* magazine and the *St. Petersburg* (Florida) *Times* newspaper turned up a series of additional Braswell legal "irregularities" that resulted in the Republican Party returning $175,000 in contributions by Braswell, as well as the return of a $100,000 Braswell campaign contribution to George W. Bush (See *St. Petersburg Times* Online, September 29, 2000).

On his last day in office as President of the United States, Bill Clinton included Braswell among the 140 felons he pardoned. It turns out that Hillary Clinton's brother, Hugh Rodham, was the attorney who actually delivered the pardon application, and was promised $230,000 if the pardon was granted. Both Bill and Hillary have denied knowing that Hugh Rodham was advocating for Braswell, and Bill Clinton has stated that he was unaware of Braswell's pending legal troubles (see *US News and World Report,* February 12, 2001).

So you have to ask yourself, "Is this who you want to buy your hair loss treatment products from?"

16

Which Hair Loss Treatment Is Right for Me?

When full-size hair transplants were still being performed, the choice of hair loss treatments was often referred to as: "drugs, rugs, or plugs." Maybe we should add "shrugs" to the list. Many people with hair loss simply choose to shrug it off as a minor issue in their life and not one worth bothering much about. But many others do indeed consider medications, or cosmetic solutions such as hairpieces, or surgery (no plugs, however).

For those who really want to do something about their hair loss there is great confusion about which method of treatment is most appropriate for their particular hair loss condition. Countless sources of information offer advice on treating hair loss, but almost all have a built-in bias toward the product or service they are selling, or by the industry or advertisers who sponsor them.

While it is no secret that I am a board certified dermatologist, and as a physician I have been prescribing medications and performing surgeries to correct hair loss for over thirty years, this chapter is an attempt to offer a balanced and useful assessment of all the treatments available for people with varying types and degrees of hair loss.

An overview of hair loss treatments is presented first, following by a listing of various types and degrees of hair loss conditions, and the most appropriate treatment options for each condition.

173

Ineffective Treatments

Doing nothing is perhaps the most common way of dealing with thinning hair. It is a completely honest solution and has no out-of-pocket cost or time requirement. This "treatment" is available to everyone with every type of hair loss. Lets face it: hair loss is not a life-threatening condition. Accepting hair loss as a natural condition is a sign of emotional security and comfort with yourself as you are.

The results, however, of doing nothing are usually unsatisfactory: Our society continues to put a high positive value on heads of healthy hair. Without treatment, the thin hair remains, and for those with androgenetic alopecia (genetic pattern hair loss), the condition usually gets worse as time goes on. While you may do just fine with thin hair or bald spots, you may also wonder how different your life would have been if you had done something about your hair loss. Sometimes the biggest risk is doing nothing at all.

But if you choose to do something about your hair loss, choose a treatment that works. Completely useless treatments are perhaps the most common way that people choose to treat their hair loss. This category includes hundreds of bizarre folk remedies, the use of "all natural" herbal lotions and scientific-sounding shampoos that claim to somehow enhance hair growth, nutritional supplements that claim to promote healthy hair, and various scalp-stimulation schemes that use electricity, LEDs, lasers, or massage to awaken the "sleeping" hair follicles. All of these treatments are, in my professional opinion as a physician, a waste of time, money, and energy. The thin hair remains, and usually gets thinner as time goes on. In addition, after the hopeful feeling wears off and the reality of the failed treatment sets in, there can be feelings of despair, frustration, anger, and often embarrassment. Furthermore, if the hair loss happens to be due to a disease condition, useless treatments may delay the person from seeking effective medical treatment, which could make the hair loss condition worse, and possibly permanent.

Cosmetic Treatments

Cosmetic treatments for hair loss are defined as methods that change the appearance but do not affect the body, and can be reversed. Hair styling, including shaving the head completely, and the use of various hair-thickening styling products are all cosmetic treatments. So are scalp paints, dust and fiber products, hairpieces and wigs, and the wearing of hats, turbans, and scarves to conceal hair loss. Cosmetic treatments range from not being very effective, to being the most effective of all the possible treatments, when measured by appearance. And just about anybody with hair loss can benefit from cosmetic treatments. Their major drawbacks are their impermanence, which brings the risk of discovery, and which requires periodic reapplications. Depending on the type of cosmetic treatment, there are varying degrees of periodic costs and time constraints as well.

Hair styling is a cosmetic treatment that most people with hair loss can benefit from. Hair frames the face, so the first consideration is to select a hairstyle that directs attention to the face, and not to the hair itself. Men with significant hair loss should avoid "comb-overs," as they tend to direct attention to the long thin strands of hair lying on top of the bald area, and do not fool the eye. To determine which styling technique will be most effective, consider the amount and quality of hair available to work with. If adequate hair exists, a permanent wave hairstyle can increase the apparent hair density by creating curls of hair that better hide the scalp. If there is little hair to work with, cutting the hair short can make a surprising improvement in appearance. Thin short hair often looks much healthier than thin long hair, which tends to fly around and lie flat. Shaving the head completely is an extreme styling technique, and for some men is works very well. Shaving the head is also a very low cost solution; however, there is the slight increased need for daily maintenance.

There are countless styling products that claim to thicken the appearance of the hair. Some conditioning products coat the hair shaft to increase thickness, while others products such as sprays, mousses, and gels help hold the hair in place. These products have limited effectiveness, but cost very little and can improve appearance to some degree. Hair coloring and bleaching products can have an effect on apparent hair density. Dyeing salt-and-pepper hair dark can in some cases make it look thicker. Alternatively, using hair coloring to make dark hair light can make it appear less thin against light colored skin. And some people find that conditioners and other products that coat the hair shaft flatten their hair and make it look thinner, and for these people avoiding styling products altogether gives their hair the fullest appearance.

Cosmetic products such as scalp paint, hair dust, and hair fiber products are ideal for temporarily increasing the apparent thickness of the hair, especially when there is no risk of someone touching it. Almost anyone with hair can increase his or her apparent hair thickness when he or she is under bright lights such as for a television appearance or an important presentation, by using these products. After the special event, you simply shampoo the product out later that evening. Hair dust and fiber products in particular can also be used immediately after transplant surgery to hide newly-placed micrografts, and allow for a very natural appearance until the grafts have healed.

The most effective of all hair restoration products are artificial hair appliances such as hairpieces and wigs, because they add the most hair and can be used by anybody with any hair loss condition. The hair used to construct these devices can be human or synthetic. For normal use, hairpieces are constructed with modest hair density so that they look natural. For movie roles, hairpieces and wigs are often constructed with more hair than would naturally occur, to give an even thicker-hair look.

Hairpieces partially cover the scalp and blend at the edges with existing hair, while wigs cover the entire scalp, including whatever hair exists. Artificial hair is ideal for those with temporary hair loss, such as hair loss from cancer treatment. Full cap wigs are often the only available solution for those with total hair loss such as from alopecia totalis, or for those with disfiguring scars on their scalp.

The main disadvantage to hairpieces and wigs is a general feeling among people that they are fake, and that they are somehow embarrassing when detected. And there is considerable maintenance time and expense involved in wearing artificial hair. The devices must be cleaned, repaired, styled and reattached on a regular basis. And artificial hair devices are delicate and begin to wear out and look unnatural after several months. They must be replaced periodically to maintain a convincing appearance. The maintenance and replacement cost of wearing a high quality hairpiece can make this option the most expensive solution for treating hair loss. Over time, the costs add up.

Wearing a hat, turban, or scarf to conceal hair loss can be a very simple, inexpensive, and effective solution, although the headgear does have to come off sometimes. People with either temporary or permanent hair loss can wear hats.

MEDICAL TREATMENTS

Medical treatments use medications to change the condition of the body and affect the hair loss condition. Medications for treating hair loss may be in the form of pills, lotions, or may be injected. Some medications block or interfere with the hormones that trigger andro-genetic alopecia. Others treat various disease conditions that include hair loss as a symptom. Preventative medications, such as Propecia and Rogaine have varying degrees of effectiveness, depending on each individual's degree of hair loss and particular body chemistry, and generally take months for a change in appearance to be notice-able. In some cases, the effect of the medication ends shortly after the drugs are discontinued. Preventative medications also require continuous use for the benefits to continue. Medications for treat-ing disease conditions also have varying degrees of effectiveness. A medicine that works very well with one person having a particular condition may have little effect on another person with the same condition. The following is a summary of five of the most commonly prescribed medications for treating hair loss: Propecia, Rogaine, spironolactone, high estrogen contraceptive pills, and corticosteroid hormone injections.

Propecia is a preventative prescription medication for men with a genetic predisposition to hair loss. Taking Propecia delays the appearance of pattern hair loss, and when treatment is started early enough, it can even help return some miniaturized hair follicles back to full size hair production. Results will vary from person to person; this is currently the best medication we have for treating male pat-tern baldness. I recommend it to most of my transplant patients as well, to help them keep the hair they have. The disadvantage of Propecia is that it is not a cure, only treatment. There is the need to take a pill once a day on a continuing basis, as well as the expense of the pills, and the very slight risk of diminished sex drive. The slight risk of diminished sex drive declines after several months use, so even if this condition occurs initially, there is a good chance it will go away after several months, or Viagra can be prescribed at ten bucks per pop to address the problem.

Minoxidil is an over-the-counter medication that is applied to the scalp to stimulate hair follicle growth, as well as to help keep active hair follicles from shutting down. Both men and women can use minoxidil lotion. It acts as "artificial life support" for hair follicles, helping to keep them producing when hormone messages or disease conditions are telling the follicles to stop producing. The results from minoxidil use vary from being very effective to not being effective at all. Like Propecia, minoxidil is a treatment and not a cure, and must be applied every day for the benefits to continue. There is a risk of scalp irritation with high concentration solutions; switching to a lower concentration usually resolves this condition.

Spironolactone is a prescription medication for women applied in lotion form to the scalp. It is prescribed for women who have a genetic predisposition for hair loss, and who have diminished female hormone levels that result in the DHT message for hair loss to finally getting through to their hair follicles. Spironolactone interferes with this message, and helps to stop the hair loss. Spironolactone is a treatment and not a cure, and must be applied every day for the benefits to continue. It also has a somewhat disagreeable odor, which can present problems in certain situations.

High estrogen oral contraceptive pills may be prescribed for women who have diminished estrogen levels and a genetic predisposition for hair loss. The estrogen in birth control pills interferes with the DHT message that is trying to tell the hair follicles to stop growing hairs. Birth control pills are a treatment and not a cure for hair loss, and the medication must be taken daily for the benefits to continue. In addition to reducing genetic hair loss, some other benefits of birth control pills include reduced risk of unwanted pregnancies, improved skin tone, reduced acne, increased bone mass, and diminished symptoms of the first stages of menopause. The risks of taking this medication on a regular basis over a long term include weight gain, increased risk of uterine cancer, increased risk of cardiovascular complications such as heart attack and stroke especially in women who smoke, and the possibility of a slightly elevated risk of breast cancer.

Corticosteroid hormone injections are a hair loss treatment that is often used for autoimmune disease conditions such as alopecia areata. Medications such as cortisone are injected directly into the patch of bald scalp to reduce the exaggerated immune response that results in white blood cells attacking the hair follicles. The effectiveness of this treatment varies, and in many cases the bald patches go away on their own, so it is difficult to determine when a particular steroid injection treatment is working or not.

Surgical Treatments

Surgical treatments for hair loss include reduction procedures where small bald portions of the scalp are removed, scalp lifts and flaps where relatively large portions of the hairy part of the scalp are rotated around to the front and top, and micrograft hair transplants where some hair follicles from the back of the scalp are moved to the front and top of the head. The results of surgical treatments usually take a few months to fully appear, however once the surgery has healed the benefits are permanent.

Scalp reductions are now most commonly used when a portion of the scalp is injured or inflamed and must be removed. It is a surgical technique where a portion of the scalp is cut out, and the edges are drawn together and closed with sutures. In the past, reduction procedures were commonly used to reduce the area needing full size grafts. They are rarely performed for this purpose today, however, because micrografting has allowed a much greater area to be effectively transplanted.

Occasionally, reduction procedures are used, along with other surgical techniques, to repair poorly-executed past hair restoration surgeries. If a patient had a transplanted hairline placed too low on the forehead, a reduction procedure could be used to pull the scalp back and raise the hairline. Reductions are also used to remove scalp tissue damaged by synthetic fiber implants. Reductions produce a permanent effect, removing a bald spot does not guarantee that the adjacent scalp won't also eventually lose hair. Reductions are simple outpatient surgical procedures performed in a doctor's office, they include the medical risks of all surgical procedures. They also leave a scar at the point where the edges of the scalp are closed. If the scalp surrounding the scar begins to lose hair, the scar may become visible. Micrografts can be transplanted directly into the scar tissue if this becomes a problem.

Scalp lifts and flap procedures are much more elaborate surgical procedures for treating hair loss, however, they are rarely performed today. With flap procedures, the patient is put to sleep under general anesthesia and sections of the bald scalp are removed, and large portions of the hairy part of the scalp are partially cut free from the scalp and rotated around to cover the open areas. The hairy flaps of scalp are stretched to cover not only the areas they had occupied, but also the areas that were covered by the bald patches of skin that were removed as well. The edges of the scalp are then sewn back together and allowed to heal. With scalp lift procedures, the entire scalp is loosened from the skull and the bald areas are removed. The hairy portions of the scalp are then stretched up and sewn together. The benefits of flap and lift procedures are the elimination of most or all of the baldness in a single visit to the surgeon. The disadvantages include the medical risks of surgery with general anesthesia, and the risk of poor cosmetic results. Although rare, patches of scalp tissue can die from inadequate blood supply after surgery, and more commonly the long scars can become visible especially as hair loss continues.

Follicular unit micrografting is the most popular form of surgical hair restoration performed today. A portion of the hair-bearing scalp from the back of the head is removed and cut into grafts containing single hairs, or naturally occurring clusters of two or more hairs. These micrografts are then placed into small slits at the front and top of the scalp, with many placed between existing hairs at the edges of the balding areas. The transplanted hair follicles are placed in a way that will give the most effective illusion of a full head of naturally growing hair. After a few months, the transplanted hair follicles begin to grow new hairs. The results are permanent, and look very natural. People who get transplants are usually thrilled with how their own hair is growing in the new location. The disadvantages include one or more outpatient surgical procedures performed in a doctor's office under local anesthetic, the considerable expense of surgery, and a small risk of poor cosmetic results, if the surgeon is inexperienced or not artistic.

17

Choosing a Physician

Choosing a hair restoration physician today is both easier than in the past, and, at the same time, more difficult. If your hair loss condition is caused by anything other than genetics, you should see a dermatologist for an examination and treatment. If your hair loss is genetic, you have a wider range of physicians to choose from.

From the 1960s through the 1980s almost all hair restoration surgical procedures and prescriptions for hair restoration medication were done by board certified dermatologists and cosmetic surgeons. Dermatologists typically performed hair transplants, scalp reductions, and prescribed medications, while cosmetic surgeons typically performed more elaborate scalp flap and scalp lift procedures. In the past, the physician selection process was fairly straightforward, and was a matter of learning about the experience and artistic abilities of the surgeon, or pharmaceutical expertise if medication was the hair restoration method desired. An initial consultation included an examination and an opportunity to see past patient photos, and ideally to meet with and examine real live past patients.

In the 1990s, a combination of two factors brought all kinds of medical doctors into the hair restoration field. The first factor was the refinement of the micrografting technique to the point where almost any physician could perform the procedure. Micrografting is considered by physicians to be a relatively simple surgical procedure that can be performed in the office. The procedure generally results in a very good to excellent outcome. Even more important, in comparison to all other forms of hair restoration surgery, micrografting has a lower risk of poor cosmetic results, as well as a low risk of medical complications. With a solid general medical training background and some specific training in micrografting techniques, micrografting made it possible for almost any medical doctor to become a hair restoration surgeon.

Also in the 1990s there was a national emphasis on cutting the cost of health care in the United States. Physicians were being financially squeezed by the cutbacks in health care, and they increasingly found their medical judgment questioned by insurance companies. Doctors and staff started spending less time with patients and more time filling out insurance forms. Some physicians believed that performing surgical procedures on patients who paid with credit cards, checks, or cash, and who really appreciated the work performed, seemed like a pleasant alternative to being questioned about tests and procedures by insurance companies and HMOs. Thousands of doctors trained in specialties ranging from heart surgery to urinary tract medicine and even pediatrics and psychiatry left those fields and entered the field of elective cosmetic surgery, including hair transplantation.

In the United States, any medical doctor can practice any type of medicine, regardless of the specific type of medical training they have had. Common sense, fear of malpractice lawsuits, and hospital qualification requirements prevent untrained doctors from performing major surgical procedures in hospital operating rooms. When a procedure is performed in the doctor's office, only common sense and fear of medical malpractice lawsuits restrict what surgical procedures are performed.

In the 1990s all areas of the elective cosmetic surgical business suddenly became much more marketing-driven than it ever had been in the past. Since the 1990s, we now have hair restoration clinics making bold advertising claims, presenting lengthy infomercials on late night cable TV, and using aggressive commission-compensated salespeople to "close deals."

Hair restoration surgery results are permanent. The hair follicles that are relocated will continue growing new hairs in the new locations for as long as they would have where they were originally located. Because micrografting is a very forgiving surgical procedure, and even a surgeon with minimal training and limited artistic abilities can achieve reasonably good results, it has become easier today than in the past to select an adequate physician to perform transplant surgery.

On the other hand, with all of the advertising hype, partial truths, and occasional false claims, is harder than ever before to find the very best physician to perform your hair restoration surgery.

The vast majority of physicians who have recently entered the field of hair restoration surgery are well-educated doctors who are capable of performing excellent micrograft transplant procedures. Some are accomplished surgeons. Many doctors have taken several days of intensive micrografting training and have worked for weeks side by side with other experienced hair restoration surgeons to learn the subtle aspects of the micrografting technique. All of these doctors are potentially excellent hair restoration surgeons. But just as is the case in any occupation, there are always a few less capable people out there. That is why it is important to take care in physician selection.

The first step in physician selection is self-education. Do as much research as you can in advance. Read books such as this one, review Internet websites, and learn about alternative treatments that may work for you. When you request information from a doctor's office, or from a clinic, you will receive literature and probably videotapes to review. The clinics will send a lot of information and will probably phone you several times as well. After doing your research, if surgery or medication, or a combination of surgery and medication seem to be the best way to address your hair loss condition, then the next step would be visiting the doctor's office for an initial consultation. Usually there is no charge for an initial consultation for hair loss restoration caused by genetics.

If you feel your hair loss is not the results of genetics, and may instead be due to a disease condition, or from a medication you are taking, or from some other cause, and you have health insurance, then you should follow the procedures for scheduling an examination that your health insurance provider recommends. You may see a primary care physician first, and after that examination, you may be referred to a dermatologist or another specialist.

Regardless of whether the doctor has been medically trained specifically to treat conditions affecting the skin and hair, or whether he or she have been trained in another medical specialty area, the examination will include an assessment of your scalp condition, over-all physical health, and emotional condition. You will be asked about any medications you are taking currently. You will be asked about any allergies to medications, such as the antibiotics and anesthetics used during surgery. It is rare that a patient comes in for hair transplants and has a health condition that would prohibit or delay surgery, but determining that possibility is one purpose of the initial exam. The doctor wants to be certain you are a qualified patient, both physically and also emotionally. A hair transplant procedure can significantly enhance your appearance, but it is not guaranteed to solve psycholog-ical problems, or make you successful in business or in relationships.

As part of the examination, your current hair loss pattern will be assessed and measured against standardized hair loss charts, such as the Hamilton/Norwood chart for men, or the Ludwig Scale for women. In addition to the pattern the character of your hair loss will also be evaluated. Is your hair thinning overall, or is it receding or forming bare bald patches? Are the remaining hairs on the top and front of your scalp very fine and short, or are they full-size and long growing? Is your hair straight or curly? Solidly colored, or salt-and-pepper? How about the donor area hairs? The character of your remaining hair, both on top and at the donor area, has a significant effect on the appearance of transplants.

The doctor will also evaluate your likely future pattern and degree of hair loss. This will be somewhat disturbing. You will face what your hair will look like decades in the future. Genetic hair loss is progressive, meaning that the degree of loss tends to increase over time. Some people lose their hair slowly, and others more rapidly, but without medical treatment, hair loss will continue year after year. The doctor will want to know about hair loss conditions of your close relatives, especially older brothers and sisters, your parents, and grandparents.

Predicting your future hair loss pattern and degree is critical not for how you will look right after transplant surgery, but rather for how you will look twenty, thirty, or forty years into the future. The most experienced and artistically capable hair restoration physicians plan their transplant procedures so that you will look natural decades into the future. This means a slightly conservative approach that includes placing some transplant grafts between existing hairs that are likely to become thin in the future, as well as avoiding a low hairline appropriate for a thirty-year old, but one that would look unnatural when the patient is in their fifties or sixties or seventies. This aspect of hair restoration surgery is more art than science, and experience counts.

Depending upon your age and current hair loss condition, the doctor may also recommend medical treatment to slow or stop your hair loss condition. A patient with a family history of extensive hair loss, who responds well to medication that stops the hair loss, is a better candidate than the same patient without the medication. Doctors who suggest medication want you to have the best possible appearance. The choice to take medication is up to you. Transplants will certainly enhance your appearance, and medication can help you keep more of the hair you have.

All of these aspects of an initial consultation and examination are reasons why it is important to meet with the doctor who will actually be doing the surgery. That is the whole point of the initial consultation. You want to be examined by the doctor who will be doing the work, and to have him or her answer your questions directly, and to allow you to answer his or her questions directly. The initial consultation is a two-way meeting, and the doctor will also ask you questions to qualify you as a patient. He or she knows what questions he or she wants answered. So be sure to get all your questions answered. Write them down, and bring them in.

Some doctors, and practically all clinics, have an "assistant" meet with you initially to determine your qualifications and to help answer some of your basic questions. These "assistants" may be medically trained personnel who also assist with the surgical procedures when not meeting prospective new patients; or they may just be salespeople. Beware of salespeople.

You will probably be asked to view a short informative video about hair restoration in general and perhaps also how that office performs the procedure specifically. You will also be able to view before-and-after photos of past patients. While these photos are impressive, keep in mind that they are typically the best results achieved. And it is difficult for someone who is not an expert to assess the effectiveness of transplant procedures from photos alone. If possible, see if you can schedule your consultation at a time when you can also meet with a past patient, so you can see the results in person for yourself.

Consider the doctor's qualifications. Look at his or her web site, if you feel uncomfortable asking the doctor about this directly. What was his or her specific area of medical training? Some doctors prominently feature the qualification "Board Certified" in their advertisements. There is no "board certification" for hair transplants. Board Certified in what field? Dermatology? Cosmetic surgery? Or maybe cardiology or urology? How long have they been performing hair restoration surgery? How many procedures have they performed?

Does the doctor have an excellent record of patient satisfaction? Some doctors subscribe to a monitoring service that randomly contacts past patients to assure that the doctor continues to keep his or her patients happy. Check the local Better Business Bureau to see if there have been complaints registered against the doctor or the clinic. If there have been complaints, have they been resolved to the patient's satisfaction? Check the state medical board to see if complaints have been registered there as well.

Finally, consider the cost of the procedure. Micrograft surgery is expensive, but the results will last a lifetime. Price is not necessarily a good measure of quality. Some inexpensive transplant clinics produce excellent results, while others produce results that look cheap. And some clinics charge very high prices, but have inexperienced or recently-trained doctors performing the actual work. The best doctors tend to charge a fair price, and you get what you pay for.

18

Future Hair Loss Treatments

Future hair loss treatments address many of the limitations of the cosmetic, medical, and surgical treatment methods currently in use, and will include some entirely new treatment methods such as hair follicle cloning and gene therapy, both of which are methods that have the potential to actually "cure" inherited pattern baldness permanently.

But it also seems reasonable to ask why human society would spend precious biomedical research effort and limited funds on hair loss treatments, when deadly and debilitating conditions such as AIDS, cancer, diabetes, and heart disease also need solutions. While economic concepts such as a "free market" and "supply and demand" are a couple of answers, it also happens that the human hair follicle is a rich scientific model for understanding important aspects of human cell biology, organ system developmental biology, immune response medicine, the process of controlled cell regeneration and differentiation, and, especially, human genetics.

A unique feature of hair follicles is the way these miniature hair-growing organs cycle through growth and rest cycles. In addition to hairs being grown and then shed in these phases, the follicle itself disintegrates almost entirely by the end of the regression phase, and an almost entirely new follicle is created at the beginning of the next growth phase. The creation of a hair follicle at the beginning of each growth phase presents unique opportunities for applying advanced molecular biology medical techniques such as cloning and gene therapy. The more we unravel the working of different parts of the human body, the more we find that everything is connected, and what we learn in one area of medicine can inevitably be applied to many other areas.

The Future of Cosmetic Treatments for Hair Loss

Cosmetic treatments for hair loss are by definition impermanent and reversible, so those aspects of cosmetic treatments will not change in the future. But other improvements will certainly be made. In the future, there will likely be hair-styling products that give a much more powerful appearance of a full head of hair, when compared to today's hair-thickening gels and hair shaft-coating mousses. Hairpieces and wigs currently have the disadvantage of expensive and time-consuming ongoing maintenance and replacement, and their use continues to include a significant fear of detection. In the future, cosmetic hair appliances such as hairpieces and wigs will likely be constructed of even finer and more durable materials, which will appear and feel even more genuine and be even less detectable. Attachment methods will continue to be very secure, but may also become easier and faster to release, reducing maintenance effort, and improving hygiene.

The Future of Medical Treatments for Hair Loss

Most of today's medicines for treating hair loss have limited effectiveness. Currently, we don't have a complete understanding of exactly why certain diseases cause hair loss. In many cases, we treat the symptoms, but not the causes of diseases. And often our ability to treat symptoms has limited effectiveness. There may be medications and treatments we are not yet aware of today that will be available in the near future. One may be treatment with a laser light apparatus or the laser comb. As of this writing, there are several reputable physicians who claim to have good results with this kind of apparatus. I have not been convinced thus far; time will tell. The same subject has been discussed with bogus treatments, Chapter 6.

Today's medications prescribed to counteract androgenetic alopecia (genetic pattern hair loss), require ongoing use for the benefits of treatment to continue, and these medications have only a limited effect on some patients. The cost of drugs, which must be taken on a continuing basis, adds up to a substantial lifetime expense. In the future, as physicians and scientists gain a better understanding of how the normal hair growth cycle is controlled and how various disease conditions affect hair growth, new medicines will be developed that more effectively target the cause of the hair loss and cause fewer side effects.

Perhaps the most promising near-future medical treatment for genetic pattern hair loss in men is GlaxoSmithKline's drug dutasteride, which as of this book's publication date has now received U.S. FDA approval as a prescription medication for treating enlarged prostate glands. Like Propecia, dutasteride is a 5-alpha-reductase inhibitor taken as a pill, and it has been shown to reduce dramatically the amount of testosterone in the blood from being converted into dihydrotestosterone (DHT). High levels of DHT in the blood over many years can cause enlarged prostate glands in men. DHT in the bloodstream also signals hair follicles to reduce hair growth, causing pattern baldness in people who have inherited hair follicles that are sensitive to DHT.

After three years of experience using dutasteride, more and more doctors are using it to treat patients who continued to lose hair when they were on Propecia. Those men who failed to stop their hair loss with Propecia, when put on Avodardt (which is dutasteride) have a greatly increased chance of stopping the balding process. Every man should be given the chance to be on finasteride (Propecia) first before transitioning to dutasteride. As stated earlier, women may well benefit from dutasteride because it effects type I alpha-reductase. No other medication we currently know of does that.

Reducing DHT in the blood causes the chemical message to "stop growing hairs" to become weaker, to a degree that it will not affect the susceptible hair follicles. The trick to reducing DHT levels is to use a medication to stop the 5-alpha-reductase enzyme from converting testosterone into DHT. If testosterone is not converted to

DHT, the DHT message never gets to the cells in the susceptible hair follicles, and these hair follicles will continue to grow new hairs.

There are two types of 5-alpha-reductase that convert testosterone to DHT. While Propecia effectively blocks the type-II 5-alpha-reductase enzyme, dutasteride has been shown to effectively block both type-I and type-II 5-alpha-reductase. While Propecia use typically results in a sixty to seventy percent decrease in DHT in the blood of men, dutasteride has been shown to decrease DHT in the blood by ninety percent or more. I am optimistic that dutasteride will work better for females with inherited pattern hair loss than any other medication currently available, as well as for men who did not get good results from Propecia. Side effects of dutasteride are believed to be similar to Propecia. The dosage appropriate for treating genetic hair loss has not been determined, and side effects are dosage-related.

One way to increase the effectiveness of hair loss medications, and simultaneously reduce side effects, is to target the cells causing hair loss. In the future we will have topical lotions applied to the scalp that more effectively block the DHT message from getting to hair follicle cells. Medications in pill form such as Propecia and dutasteride affect DHT levels in the blood, which in turn affects the amount of DHT in scalp tissue, which in turn affects DHT concentrations at the cellular level in hair follicles. As a result of treating the entire system with the medication, unwanted side effects can occur in areas other than the hair follicle cells.

In the future we will be able to better affect the DHT levels in the cells in the hair follicles, and as a result better control hair loss, and reduce unwanted side effects. Maybe medications of the future will be combined with shampoos or hair conditioners, and these products will become a common way to keep hair from falling out, just as fluoride in toothpaste is now used to help prevent teeth from falling out.

There will also be advances in medications for treating hair loss conditions other than genetic pattern hair loss. In the future we will develop new drugs that will more powerfully signal certain cells in the hair follicles to start or remain in the anagen (growing) phase, and continue to grow hair, even when they get other signals to shut down, such as from sudden stressful events. And we will make advances in medications for treating diseases that cause both temporary and permanent hair loss.

Diseases and conditions that cause temporary hair loss are called non-scarring alopecias by doctors. These diseases do not seem to harm or scar the hair follicle in a permanent way. The hair is lost, but it either regrows all by itself, or with the right chemical signals, can be made to regrow. Alopecia areata is a non-scarring alopecia. Some alopecia areata patients have been able to regrow hair even after years of constant hair loss. Hair loss resulting from chemotherapy, and moderate doses of radiation treatment, are also non-scarring. Hair shafts that are pulled or plucked from the follicle do not permanently damage the follicle. After being plucked, the follicle rests and recovers, and a new hair bulb is grown, and it then grows a new hair.

Non-scarring alopecias affect the "bulb" portion of the hair follicle, which is located at the base of the follicle deep in the skin. The specialized cells in the bulb do the work of growing the hair shaft for four to six years during each hair growth cycle, but at the end of the growth cycle they seem to deteriorate as the hair follicle shrinks in size and enters the resting stage of the normal growth cycle. New hair follicle bulb cells are then produced at the beginning of the subsequent growth cycle. Future medications that effectively target or protect the cells in the bulb of the hair follicle may result in more effective treatment for alopecia areata, as well as less hair loss from stressful events and cancer treatments.

Diseases that cause permanent hair loss are called scarring alopecias, because the disease alters or scars the hair follicle in such a way that it loses the ability to grow new hairs. Some scarring alopecias, such as lupus erythematosus and lichen planopilaris, trigger an inflammatory immune response where the body's white blood cells attack cells in the "bulge" area of the hair follicle. The bulge area is located near the middle of the hair follicle, below the sebaceous (oil) gland and near the attachment point for the arrector pili muscle (the tiny muscle that allows hairs to "stand on end").

Androgenetic alopecia (genetic pattern hair loss) is also considered to be a scarring alopecia, as it diminishes hair follicle production over time until no new hairs are grown. New research has suggested the area of inflammation in these permanent hair loss diseases is the "bulge" portion of the hair follicle, and certain cells in the bulge area are believed to be responsible for regrowing the hair follicle at the beginning of each new growth stage. It is believed that at the beginning of each growth stage, certain cells in the bulge produce the cells in the bulb, which in turn grow new hairs. When the cells in the bulge area are sufficiently injured, the hair follicle is not able to grow a new bulb, and no new hair is produced. In the future, medications that protect the cells in the bulge area of the hair follicle will more effectively treat permanent hair loss diseases, including genetic pattern hair loss.

The Future of Surgical Treatments for Hair Loss

Surgical treatments available today are limited in effectiveness because no new hair is added. Current surgical methods simply cannot produce a full head of thicker hair. The art of surgical hair restoration is rearranging the patient's existing DHT-resistant hair follicles for an appearance that looks fuller. But no new hair is added. Current surgical methods are very labor intensive and costly, and include the minor discomfort of recovery following surgery. The obvious key to improving surgical treatment is cloning hair follicles. Successfully cloning multiple hair follicles from a donor area follicle that is already programmed to continue to grow new hairs for a lifetime will result in a limitless supply of hair transplant grafts, which translates into limitless hair thickness. The cloned follicles may even be individually injected directly into the scalp, eliminating surgery altogether.

If scientists can already clone an entire sheep, why isn't human hair follicle cloning a commercial reality? The answer is somewhat complicated, and requires some explanation of cell biology, genetics, cell replication, and then a review of some of the different types of cloning that may apply in the future to mass duplication of human hair follicles.

Cell Biology

Cells are the basic units of all living organisms. Cells in a multi-celled organism have specialized characteristics that enable them to most efficiently do their particular jobs. Individual cells in an organism work together with other similar cells in tissue, or they work together with different types of cells in specialized cell structures called organs. For example, in a hair follicle, which is a miniature organ, there are several different types of cells working together to grow a hair.

Inside of just about every mature cell is a structure called a cell nucleus that contains chromosomes composed of double strands of twisted DNA molecules. DNA molecules contain information about creating particular types of proteins, and the cell uses that information to make the proteins that allow it to perform its particular function. Some proteins are structural, such as keratin protein in hair, while others have the function of sending messages, such as the hormone DHT, and some proteins such as the enzyme 5-alpha-reductase, help convert proteins from one form to another.

Genetics

Sections of DNA molecules that contain the code for particular types of proteins are called genes. That's all genes are: instructions for making specific proteins. There are no genes for particular body characteristics—such as "pattern baldness" or "green eyes" or "curly hair"—only instructions for making proteins. But the particular types of proteins that genes instruct cells to make, in turn determine characteristics such as inherited hair loss and eye color and hair curling. Usually many different genes, and many different proteins, together determine particular inherited body characteristics.

Unlocking the DNA information in mature specialized cells is an important aspect of some cloning techniques. This is because a remarkable feature of cells in a multi-celled organism is that each one contains in its chromosomes a complete DNA blueprint of all the genes for all the proteins for the entire organism. In theory, any cell from an organism could be used to clone the entire organism. But actually doing this with a mature specialized cell is very difficult. Individual cells only use the protein-making information that they need to do their particular job, even though they contain the protein-making information for the entire organism. For example, cells in the iris of the eye may make the proteins that express the characteristics for green eyes, but not the proteins that could cause pattern baldness or curly hair. The information to make proteins that result in pattern baldness or curly hair is contained in the iris cells. They just don't express those proteins. Other cloning techniques require unspecialized cells called stem cells for the desired results. To understand the difference between using mature specialized cells or stem cells from cloning, we need to examine the process of cell replication.

CELL REPLICATION

In a rapidly growing embryo, cells replicate by splitting in half and then growing to full size again. This process is called cell mitosis, and each half of a cell that splits containing a complete and exact set of the organism's DNA. As the embryo grows into a more fully functioning organism, its cells begin to take on more specialized characteristics, and begin to divide less. As cells become more specialized, cell replication shifts to special precursor cells called stem cells.

Mature specialized cells do not replicate easily, probably as a defense against cancer, which is characterized by uncontrolled cell division. But all cells wear out over time, and have to be replaced by new cells. Some cells only last for days; others for years, and others for decades, but eventually all cells wear out. The inability of mature cells to replicate themselves limits the body's ability to repair itself, to heal wounds and to replace aging cells. It also makes the process of cloning more difficult.

In mature organisms, undifferentiated cells called stem cells are responsible for replacing old or injured specialized cells. Stem cells are present in all self-repairing tissue, but most stem cells are difficult to detect in a mature living organism. Stem cells in a mature organism are like embryonic cells, in that they can create many different types of specialized cells. When stem cells are not actively making new cells, they divide infrequently, which reduces the risk of undesirable DNA mutations. But when they are signaled to make new cells of a particular type, they produce typically short-lived intermediate cells called transient amplifying cells, which in turn engage in rapid cell mitosis and create the specialized cells that the organism needs.

For a quick review, we've learned that cells make up tissue and organs, which make organisms. The DNA in cells contains genes that are instructions for making proteins, and these proteins determine specialized cell characteristics and functions. Specialized cells in turn, determine characteristics of an organism, including inherited characteristics, such as resistance to the hormone DHT, for example. Specialized cells do not easily replicate themselves. When an organism needs new specialized cells, stem cells are signaled to create transient amplifying cells, which in turn make the needed specialized cells.

Types of Cloning

Cloning is the process of reproducing cells, organs, or entire organisms from a single parent, in contrast to sexual reproduction, which involves the mixing of DNA from both parents. Cloning results in offspring that have an exact copy of the DNA of the single parent. This is desirable if the parent's DNA has desirable characteristics, such as hair follicle cells resistance to DHT. There are many different types of cloning that may apply to hair follicles, including the DNA manipulation type that produced Dolly the Sheep; the "splitting hairs" method; the process of replicating mature cells; and growing new organs from stem cells. Each of these four methods will be described and evaluated as a possible basis for commercial hair follicle cloning.

Dolly the Sheep Cloning Method

In 1997, Dolly the Sheep became the most famous cloned animal. DNA was removed from an unfertilized donor sheep egg cell, and then was replaced with DNA from a mature cell removed from Dolly's parent. An unfertilized egg has only half of the DNA needed to grow into an organism. The other half comes from the sperm cell. But Dolly's egg received a full set of DNA from a mature cell. The egg was fooled into thinking it was fertilized, and that it should grow into an organism. The egg cell grew into an embryo, and eventually into a sheep that was an exact genetic copy of Dolly's parent, since it had the exact same DNA. This was the first time a large mammal was grown from DNA taken from a mature cell, using that cell's entire DNA blueprint to make a new organism. The process is much more involved than this summary describes, and there were many failures along the way. But if we just want some hair follicles, cloning an entire living organism from a donor cell is a bit excessive. While a fascinating genetic exercise, the Dolly the Sheep method is too complicated and costly for commercial hair follicle cloning. Another method, which is inadvertently used in almost every micrograft hair transplant procedure, is a lot easier.

THE SPLITTING HAIRS METHOD OF CLONING

Hair restoration surgeons have long known about the "splitting hairs" method of cloning hair follicles, and it is a much less complicated process than the Dolly the Sheep method. Surgeons have observed that when a hair follicle is accidentally cut in half, one piece,

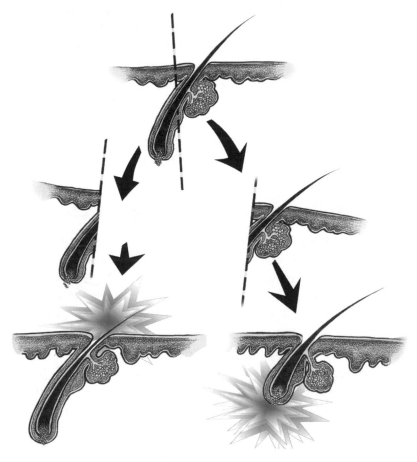

Cloning follicles by "splitting hairs"

and sometimes both pieces of the follicle, will survive and grow a new hair if the follicle is transplanted back into the donor. Micrograft surgeons routinely place cut follicles back into the patient's scalp, although they don't generally "count" the cut follicles as "grafts." Each fractional follicle is an exact DNA clone of the original, so if the original follicle is DHT-resistant, the clones will also be DHT-resistant.

If a follicle is cut in half to form top and bottom pieces, and both pieces are placed back in the scalp, the bottom half (with the hair bulb) will sometimes survive and grow a hair. The top half (with the bulge) will sometimes survive and grow a new bottom half containing a new hair bulb, and that half also eventually grows a new hair. This process is similar to the hair follicle creation that occurs at the beginning of the normal hair follicle growth phase. If the follicle is cut lengthwise, two surviving follicles can result, although they may produce finer hairs than the original full-size follicle.

Survival rates of transected hair follicles is lower than follicles that are not cut in half, so hair restoration surgeons continue to take great care to avoid cutting follicles. The reason the splitting hairs methods works when the cut follicle pieces are placed back into the scalp, is that other nearby hair follicle stem cells probably help with the cell regeneration process. But with improved methods to signal cell regeneration, and ultimately improved transected follicle survival rates, this crude cloning technique has some promise for the immediate future.

MATURE CELL CLONING

Commercially cloning of undifferentiated stem cells for research purposes has been around for a few years. Recently the commercialization of cloning mature skin cells has been accomplished. On June 20, 2000 the U.S. FDA approved Organogenesis Incorporated's Apligraf, a skin patch product containing living human skin cells. To make an Apligraf patch, human skin cells derived from infant foreskins are cultured in a growth medium and are allowed to differentiate into some of the types of cells that form mature human skin. Apligraf skin does not contain pigment cells, blood vessels, sweat glands, or hair follicles, but it does have the types of cells that are typically found in the upper and lower layers of skin. It is approved for use as a wound dressing for slow healing skin ulcers.

Replicating skin cells is much less complicated than replicating entire hair follicles. The approval and commercialization of this mature cell cloning process is very encouraging for future hair follicle cloning. Because hair follicles are miniature organs composed of several different types of specialized cells, they are difficult to clone and even more difficult to assemble properly. The trick to hair follicle cloning will be signaling hair follicle stem cells to make and assemble all the cells needed for a hair follicle.

In 1993, United Kingdom researchers Jahoda and Reynolds published a paper in *The Journal of Investigative Dermatology* describing their success in growing a rat whisker in a live rat from cultured rat dermal papilla cells. The dermal papilla cells are found in the hair matrix in the bulb of the hair shaft, and they are the cells that grow hairs. For many years it was believed that the hair follicle bulb contained the stem cells necessary for hair follicle growth. The researchers removed dermal papilla cells from a rat whisker hair follicle bulb, cultured the cells in a growth medium, and created thousands of dermal papilla cell clones. After they had enough dermal papilla cells, they implanted the cultured cells back into the rat, but they placed the cells in the skin forming the rat's ear (so they could better see any results). The cloned dermal papilla cells interacted with neighboring skin cells and made a hair follicle that eventually grew a rat whisker. The researchers patented this procedure of growing hair follicles in a living organism with cloned dermal papilla cells. (Jahoda and Reynolds, *Journal of Investigative Dermatology* (101:634-638, 1993) (also 115:587-593, 1992)

In 1994, *The Journal of Dermatological Science* published a paper by the same researchers, Jahoda and Reynolds, describing their success using a cell culture medium to grow a crude but functioning rat hair follicle from cultured adult hair follicle cells. The researchers cultured four different types of cells found in rat hair follicles, and using a framework of other living cells, assembled them into somewhat unusual hair bulb structures that grew irregular but recognizable hair shafts. This appears to be the first example of growing "test tube" hair follicles outside of a living organism.

In 1996, hair restoration surgeon Jerry Cooley, MD successfully grew human hair follicles from cloned dermal papilla cells in a human. He cultured dermal papilla cells from hair follicle bulbs surgically removed from his own scalp, and after multiplying the cells in a culture medium, implanted the cloned cells back into his own forearm, and a new hair follicle formed and grew a scalp hair.

In 1998, Dr. Conradus Ghosal Gho of the Netherlands patented with the World Intellectual Property Organization, a "Method for the Propagation of Hair", in which he describes a method of plucking hairs in the anagen (growth) phase, and culturing the dermal papilla cells from the portion of the hair bulb at the end of the plucked hair. He describes using commercial cell culture media along with various beneficial additives such as amino acids, vitamins, trace elements, growth hormones, and antibiotics. His patent seems to imply that the best results are achieved by also adding cloned CD34+ progenitor cells, a type of stem cell, to the culture. Presumably these would be obtained by surgically removing a tissue sample from the donor, and culturing the stem cells separately, so they could be added to the dermal papilla cell culture. Alternatively, the CD34+ cells may be obtained commercially. After the dermal papilla cells and CD34+ cell mixture has multiplied and differentiated into the different types of cells that make up hair follicle, Dr Gho injects packets of the cloned cell mixture into the donor's scalp, where they develop into new hair follicles and grow new hairs. Dr. Gho also describes using an electronic repeating injection metering apparatus such as an insulin pen to rapidly and precisely insert the cloned cells into the scalp. Dr. Gho is currently working to refine and improve his method.

It seems that it won't be long before cloning thousands of whole human hair follicles in "test tubes" becomes a commercial reality. Or will it? There are still plenty of obstacles to overcome before commercial hair follicle cloning is a reality. The method of cloning dermal papilla cells from hair bulbs and injecting them back into the donor's scalp has not been perfected. Do the hair follicles created from cultured dermal papilla cells cycle through the normal growth cycles, and continue to grow new hairs for a lifetime? What are the chemical signals in living skin that tell the dermal papilla cells to grow into a hair follicle in the first place? If we knew more about how the hair follicle growth cycle functioned, maybe we could improve the results of injecting cloned cells to make hair follicles. Or perhaps we could clone cells into entire hair follicles in "test tubes" and achieve better results than injecting packets of cloned cells.

The Wall Street Journal May 4, 2005 had an article on hair cloning in which they stated Dr. Unger of Toronto and Dr. Gho of the Netherlands both have patents on hair cloning and although it has worked in mice, "It's likely to be years before someone as bald as actor Bruce Willis will be able to walk into a doctor's office, donate a few hairs for multiplying, return for scalp injections ten days later and end up with a full head of hair in a matter of months."

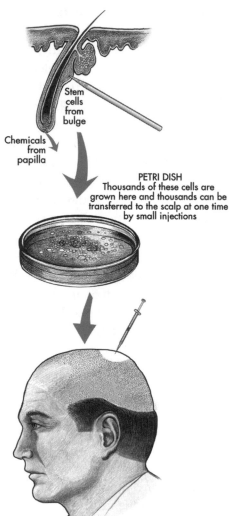

Stem cells from bulge

Chemicals from papilla

PETRI DISH
Thousands of these cells are grown here and thousands can be transferred to the scalp at one time by small injections

More answers to the future of hair follicle cloning appear in work done over the last decade by Dr. Robert Lavker and his associate Dr. George Cotsarelis, both of the Department of Dermatology at he University of Pennsylvania School of Medicine.

In a paper published in 1990 in the journal *Cell,* Cotsarelis showed that hair follicle stem cells were located in the bulge area of the follicle, midway up the hair shaft, rather than in the bulb area at the base of the hair shaft. The bulge area is located near the middle of the hair follicle, below the sebaceous (oil) gland and near the attachment point for the arrector pili muscle (the tiny muscle that allows hairs to "stand on end").

The April 2004 issue of *Nature Biotechnology* published research findings from the University of Pennsylvania School of Medicine that had isolated stem cells responsible for hair follicle growth within the follicle bulge. In studies involving adult mice, transplanted stem cells made new hair follicles that produced new hair within four weeks. According to research director Cotsarelis, isolating the stem cells responsible for hair growth—which are there throughout the lifespan of an organism and have tremendous capacity to regenerate and proliferate—is the first step to developing targets for manipulating hair growth. Researchers at the Penn Hair and Scalp Clinic hope to eventually isolate stem cells in adult humans and transplant those cells to other areas of the scalp, generating new follicles and hair growth, but the treatment is a good ten years away.

On behalf of the Trustees of the University of Pennsylvania, Lavker has registered several patents for methods for regulating hair growth. In a 1996 patent filed with the World Intellectual Property Organization (and cited by Dr. Gho in his patent two years later), Lavker describes a hair follicle bulge activation theory, in which the dermal papilla cells activate the stem cells in the bulge in the late telogen (resting) stage of hair growth. This is the point at which the dermal papilla cells move upwards and next to the bulge area of the follicle, after the follicle has shed the old hair and has shrunk in size. Once the stem cells are activated, a new hair follicle growth cycle begins, the follicle grows to full size, and a new hair bulb forms to grow a new hair.

Lavker states that the hair matrix cells are in fact transient amplifying cells; intermediate cells created by stem cells to rapidly grow other specialized cells, in this case those that make up a hair shaft. The 1996 patent describes growth-modulating molecules that are created by hair follicle cells and which undergo hair-cycle-dependent concentration changes in the hair follicle. One such molecule is a protein called glia-derived nexin 1, which has also been shown to play important roles in regulating a variety of types of cellular growth and differentiation.

Lavker's 1996 patent claims applications in modulating hair growth, as well as for growing hair follicle cells outside of a body with a selected growth-modulating molecule, and combining the expanded cells with selected dermal papilla cells to grow hair.

In a year 2000 paper published in *Dermatology Focus,* Cotsarelis reveals that he is working on cloning hair follicle stem cells in cultures, and that once the molecular events responsible for the cycle of hair follicle growth is unraveled, cloning entire hair follicles will be closer to reality.

This research suggests that the most likely method for commercial hair follicle cloning is not cloning dermal papilla cells, but the cloning of hair follicle stem cells collected from the bulge area of DHT-resistant hair follicles. These stem cells will be combined with proteins that provide the right molecular signals to tell the stem cells to generate transient amplifying cells in the form of a hair bulb, which in turn will grow a new hair.

Once these details are figured out, thousands of full-size "test-tube" grown hair follicles can be self-assembled from cloned DHT resistant stem cells. The cloned hair follicles could be grown in a standard size and shape, perhaps in a tray that can be directly loaded into an automatic graft placement device. Automated graft placement devices, such as Choi Transplanter developed by Yung Chul Choi, MD in Korea in 1990, use a hollow needle to create a tiny recipient site of the proper depth for the graft, and then automatically insert the graft into the opening.

There will still be some problems associated with cloning. One is an increased risk of cancer. The growth-inducing chemicals such as tetradecanoylphorbol acetate (TPA) used to stimulate cellular proliferation for cloning frequently promote tumors and cancer. While cancer risk is low for most cloned cell products, cloning hair follicle stem cells is riskier.

Dermatologists have observed that many basal cell carcinomas, a type of skin cancer that is the most common human tumor, seem to originate from the hair follicle. Cotsarelis notes in the 2000 paper presented in *Dermatology Focus:* "...the fact that basal cell carcinomas are slow-growing tumors composed of poorly differentiated cells that have the ability to differentiate into various adnexal structures strongly suggests that the cell of origin is a pluripotent, slowly cycling stem cell with a highly proliferative potential." What he's saying is that molecular and genetic evidence points to the hair follicle stem cell as the source for this common form of cancer. Cloning hair follicle stem cells with cancer-inducing chemicals will require many years of study to assure the safety of the cloned follicles that result.

HAIR MULTIPLICATION— SCALP IMPREGNATION THERAPY

This cell based, tissue engineered treatment for hair loss is touted as the "Holy Grail" of hair restoration. The term "hair multiplication" was coined by Dr. Gho of the Netherlands. In theory, this minimally invasive high tech surgical procedure should deliver an unlimited supply of donor hair to the patient. Hair cells are extracted from a small donor site in the scalp, then cultured and multiplied in a lab. Balding areas are then replanted with the cultured cells suspension. Dr. Carl Bazan of Mexico offers hair multiplication under the proprietary name "Scalp Impregnation Therapy." A twenty-minute impregnation session—administering cultured hair cells suspension quantified in ounces—claims to yield up to 6,000 hairs with negligible discomfort. As with any new medical breakthrough, the results are yet undetermined and cost for treatment is high—ranging from $22,000 to 36,000.

Research conducted by Colin Jahoda of the University of Durham in England in the early 1990s demonstrated that the cells at the base of a follicle can and do regenerate into self-contained, pre-programmed hair factories. These cells mature into hair follicles through a process known as *follicular neogenesis*. In theory, if this technology can be perfected, it will solve the supply and demand scalp-harvesting problem. To date, however, Dr. Gho's experiments find only twenty percent of implanted cells maturing into follicles.

Interesting to note, the molecules responsible for telling a hair to grow are in the same family of molecules that tell the liver, the kidney, or even a full limb to grow. If science can figure out exactly what turns on the regeneration of hair follicles, the field of tissue engineering will be advanced and science may one day be able to help an amputee grow a new limb.

Dr. Walter Unger recently presented information regarding an ongoing study on culturing hair matrix cells to produce unlimited donor hair. His work with Dr. D. N. Sauder to discover what is required to culture and reimplant hair matrix cells has shown that they can now be produced fairly rapidly for all patients. They will be doing studies on the cultured cells in mice and hope to start testing in humans, but this will require ethical permission from the governing medical boards. Likely this will be available to the public in ten years time.

Gene Therapy

An even more advanced technique for solving inherited hair loss in the future is gene therapy. Gene therapy is the process of changing genes of existing cells in the body, and thereby altering cell function. It is a medical treatment still in its infancy, and there have only been a few recent examples of gene therapy working. But it is a potential future baldness treatment method worth exploring.

Gene therapy requires learning how an inherited medical condition occurs at the DNA molecule level, and then going in and fixing it. With gene therapy, the hair follicles with DHT-sensitive cells could be changed into follicles with DHT-resistant cells, and the hair follicles would continue to grow new hairs for a lifetime. But gene therapy involves several very difficult steps. The first step is figuring out which of the tens of thousands of genes on strands of DNA are involved in the characteristic to be altered, and the second step is figuring out how exactly the target genes are to be changed, so that they give instructions for making the slightly different proteins that will achieve the desired effect. The third step is getting the target cells in the living organism to incorporate the new and improved genes as replacements for the old undesirable genes.

Gene Identification

Figuring out which genes are involved in the genetic condition to be changed is not an easy task. Despite all the advances in mapping genes in recent years, we are still very far away from knowing what most of these genes do. We certainly do not have a good understanding of all of the genes that affect the cycle of hair growth, and especially which genes are responsible for inherited hair loss. It is most likely that several genes are responsible for making proteins that cause certain hair follicles to be DHT-sensitive.

Future studies will likely involve comparing the genes and resulting proteins in different follicles from a single individual. In a given individual with androgenetic alopecia (pattern hair loss), some hair follicle cells will express the characteristic of DHT-resistance (the follicles at the back of the scalp), while other hair follicles on the same person will express the characteristic of DHT-sensitivity (at the hairline, for example). Both follicles contain cells with identical DNA, but they express different characteristics. So identifying the responsible genes will be tricky. And even after we identify these genes, we have to figure out how to change them ever so slightly so they will make proteins that create DHT-resistant hair follicles.

Scientists have been making progress in gene identification. To identify genes that may participate in a given response, gene arrays profiling is used to determine the genes that are differentially expressed. To use this molecular knowledge for enhancing protection and repair, it is necessary to over express the genes of choice. Future identification of genes that are important for protection and regeneration, along with improved gene transfer technology, will allow the use of gene therapy for treating a wide range of hereditary disease.

MODIFYING GENES

In a paper presented in the January 30, 1998 issue of the journal *Science,* researchers led by Angela Christiano PhD., identified a defect in a single gene responsible for a rare type of inherited baldness called generalized atrichia observed in a Pakistani family, in which affected individuals are born with infant hair that falls out and never grows back. Shortly after birth, affected individuals are completely hairless. The gene, called *hairless,* was mapped in humans to chromosome 8p21, and was the first example of a single gene defect being identified as a hair loss cause. Christiano was careful to point out that this was just a first step towards identifying genes that affect hair loss. (*Science,* January 30,1998, Vol. 279, No. 5351)

Later in the same year, in a paper presented in the September 11, 1998 issue of *The American Journal of Human Genetics,* Christiano's team reported on members of a family of Irish Travelers who also exhibited congenital atrichia, in which affected individuals are born with infant hair that falls out and never grows back. Genetic analysis of the Irish Travelers revealed that a mutation of the hairless gene was again responsible for the hair loss condition. The mutation, however, was different from the one that resulted in hair loss in the Pakistani family.

In a paper reported in the November 25 1998 issue of *Cell,* researchers led by Elaine Fuchs PhD, induced the formation of new hair follicles in mice that were genetically engineered to constantly produce a stabilized form of a protein called beta-catenin. Beta-catenin is a multi-functional protein which signals a variety of cellular functions, but is normally quickly degraded within a cell after being produced. Researchers altered the mouse gene that contains instructions for making the beta-catenin protein in such a way that the beta-catenin produced was resistant to being broken down. The resulting accumulation of beta-catenin caused a massive growth of new hair follicles to grow in normal mouse skin, until there were hair follicles branching from existing hair follicles. Eventually the mice also developed hair follicle tumors as a result of over-expressing beta-catenin. (Fuchs, University of Chicago 1998) (Gat, *Dermatology Focus* Vol. 19, No. 2, Summer 2000).

In the October 1999 issue of *The Journal of Clinical Investigation,* researchers led by Dr. Ronald Crystal forced resting hair follicles of mice into the growth phase by exposing cells to larger than normal quantities of a protein produced by the Sonic Hedgehog Gene (abbreviated Shh).

The papers presented by these three groups of genetic researchers reveal the complexity of the task of understanding the genetic basis for inherited hair loss, and reveal the monumental task of figuring out how to correct the condition at the molecular level. In the first case, Angela Christiano's team identified a gene that can cause total hair loss when mutated in either of two different ways. In the second example, the team led by Elaine Fuchs mutated a gene in such a way that it coded for the creation of a slightly different protein that caused massive new hair follicle creation. And the third example showed that increasing the exposure to a naturally occurring protein could signal hair follicles to shift from the resting phase into the growth phase. And while all of these genes and their respective proteins appear to play some role in hair follicles, they are also known to affect other cells and systems in the body. Genetics is very complicated.

But suppose that at some point in the future we develop an adequately complete understanding of how all the genes, and their respective proteins, affect inherited hair loss. And suppose that we can also determine how exactly we want to alter the genes so that the proteins they make result in hair follicles that are DHT-resistant, rather than DHT-sensitive, but without causing unwanted side effects.

Changing Genes in Living Cells and Living Organisms

The third challenge of gene therapy is delivering the new-and-improved genes to the target cells, and then to have those cells use the new genes to make the corresponding new proteins, and then to have the altered cells express the desired characteristic.

The correct target cells are critical to successful gene therapy. If mature cells are altered, the benefits of the gene therapy go away after those cells wear out and are replaced with new cells having the original DNA. For a long-lasting effect, stem cells are targeted. When successful, the altered stem cells will then create altered transient amplifying cells, which in turn will create altered specialized cells that will express the desired characteristics.

The most common altered gene-delivery method involves using crippled viruses to insert desired genes into the target cells. Outside of the laboratory, viruses are tiny organisms that infect cells by replacing some of the cell's DNA with virus DNA. After infection by a virus, a cell begin to make the proteins the virus DNA tells it to make, causing the expression of various diseases. Scientists use the virus infection mechanism to deliver desirable DNA.

First, they cripple the virus DNA so that it cannot reproduce or cause harmful effects, but is still able to insert new DNA into target cells. The desired genes are spliced onto to the virus DNA, and the viruses insert the new DNA into the target cells. The viruses can be injected directly to the location where the stem cells are, or the stem cells may be cultured in a laboratory, altered by viruses containing the new DNA, and then the altered stem cells can be placed back into the organism.

There are many areas of gene therapy that need refinement. Identifying genes, determining exactly how to change them to code for the desired proteins, avoiding an immune response when the viruses are injected directly into the organism, getting an adequate quantity of target cells to take up the altered DNA regardless of how it is delivered, and getting the cells to express the characteristics coded by the altered genes, once the new DNA is inserted, all need more work. But progress is being made.

In summary, the future of hair loss treatment shows great promise, from new medications such as dutasteride to advances in cloning and gene therapy. But many of these treatments are years, and maybe decades away from commercial use. Current treatment methods, including cosmetic products, drugs such as Propecia, and surgical procedures such as follicular unit micrografts are available right now, if you really want to do something about your hair loss. Your first step should be scheduling an examination with a dermatologist knowledgeable about hair loss treatment.

APPENDIX 1:

Sources for More Information

- American Academy of Dermatology
  1567 Maple Ave
  Evanston IL 60201
  312-869-3954
  www.aad.com
  (Information on dermatology, including hair loss.)

- American Academy of Cosmetic Surgery
  159 East Live Oak Ave #204
  Arcadia CA 91006
  818-447-1579
  www.cosmeticsurgery.org
  (Information on various hair restoration procedures.)

- American Society for Dermatologic Surgery
  5550 Meadowbrook Dr. Suite 120
  Rolling Meadows, IL 60008
  847-956-0900
  www.asds-net.org
  (A good source for dermatologic and hair restoration surgeons)

- American Hair Loss Council
  100 Independence Place #207
  800-274-8717
  www.ahlc.org
  (Good source for hairpiece and wig information.)

- International Society of Hair Restoration Surgery
  www.ishrs.com
  (Source for hair restoration surgeons worldwide)

- National Alopecia Areata Foundation
  PO Box 5027
  Mill Valley CA 94911
  415-383-34444
  www.naaf.org
  (Best source for alopecia areata information)

- www.hairdoc.com
  2001 Union Street #520
  San Francisco, Ca. 94123
  415-922-3344
  (A good source for unbiased up-to-date information on hair loss)

- International Alliance of Hair Restoration Surgeons
  www.iahrs.org
  (Good source to find hair restoration surgeons.)
  www.regrowth.com
  (Information on medical treatments for hair loss.)
  www.thebaldtruth.com
  (Good source for all types of hair loss treatments.)

- www.quackwatch.com
  (Reveals all types of medical scams, including bogus hair loss treatments.)

Appendix 2
Drugs That Can Cause Hair Loss

The following sources were used to create this list of drugs that can cause hair loss, however the list is still far from comprehensive.

1. *Drug Eruption Reference Manual, Eleventh Edition,* Litt, Jerome Z. Taylor and Francis

2. *Dermatology Moschella and Hurley,* Moschella, Samuel L., Hurley, Harry J. (eds) WB Saunders Company, Philadelphia 1985

3. *Disorders of Hair Growth,* Olsen, Elise A. (ed) McGraw Hill Inc. New York 1994

4. *Clinical Dermatology,* 2nd Edition, Habif, Thomas P. CV Mosby Company, St. Louis 1990

5. *Diseases of the Hair and Scalp,* Rook A, Dawber RPR (eds) Blackwell Scientific Publications, Oxford 1991

6. *Hair Loss: Principles of Diagnosis and Management of Alopecia,* Shapiro, Jerry, Martin Dunitz, London 2002

Most of the listed drugs have multiple names, including generic names and often many brand names. Brand names for medications can vary from country to country. Every name for every drug is not included in the list.

It is important to note that the incidence of hair loss occurring from the vast majority of these drugs is infrequent, often only one to two percent of users, and when it does occur is usually happens only after prolonged use of the medication. Many common medications are listed as possibly causing hair loss. They do not usually cause hair loss in most people, but have been documented to cause hair loss in some people.

Some drugs that are prescribed to help grow hair or slow hair loss, such as minoxidil, spironolactone, and oral contraceptives, are also included in this list of drugs that cause hair loss. This is not a mistake, but rather illustrates the complex ways that bodies respond to medications. And sometimes these drugs initially trigger hair shedding which is followed by increased hair growth.

If you are taking any of the listed medications and suspect that one or more may be causing your hair loss, discuss your concern with your physician. You may also wish to do some additional research on the drug or drugs you are concerned about. Your physician may determine that it is possible to switch to an alternative medication. In most cases, hair growth resumes after the medication that caused the hair loss is discontinued.

The numbers in parenthesis after each listed drug indicates the source or sources listing that drug as a possible cause of hair loss. Some of these reference guides in turn list studies published in medical journals describing the occurrence and frequency of side effects such as hair loss.

One class of medications cause hair loss in nearly 100 percent of patients within a week or two after taking the drugs. Thesse

A new feature of this edition of this book is the listing of brand names. The generic names are in the left column and the most common brand name on the right column.

Generic name	**Brand name**
A	
Acebutolol (1)	Sectral
Acetaminophen (1)	Tylenol
Acetohexamide (1)	Dymelor
Acitretin (1) (5) (6)	Soriatane
Acyclovir (1)	Zovirax
Actinomycin-D (1) (5)	Cosmegen
Albendazole (1) (3)	Albenza
Aldesleukin (1)	Proleukin
Alfa Interferons (1)	
Alitretinoin (1)	Panretin
Allopurinol (1) (2) (3) (4) (5)	Zyloprim
Altretamine (1)	Hexalen
Amamtadine (1)	Symmetrel
Amiloride (1)	Midamor
Aminophylline (1)	
Aminosalicylate sodium (1)	Paser Granules
Amiodarone (1) (5)	Pacerone

Amitriptyline (1)..Elavil
Amlodipine (1).. Norvasc
Amphotericin B (1) .... Amphocin
Anagrelide (1) ....Agrylin
Anastrozole (1) .... Arimidex
Androstenedione (1) .... Androstene
Anisindione (1) .... Miradon
Anthrax Vaccine (1)..................Anthrax Vaccine Adsorbed (AVA)
Aprepitant (1) .... Emend
Aripiprazole (1)..Abilify
Arsenic (1)..Trisonex
Asparaginase (1) (6) .... **Elspar**
Aspirin (1)
Atazanavir (1)..Reyataz
Atenolol (1) ....Tenoretic
Atorvastatin (1).. Lipitor
Azathioprine (1) (5) ....Imuran

B

Balsalazide (1) ....Colazal
Bendroflumethiazide (1)..Corzide
Benzphetamine (1) .... Didrex
Betaxolol (1) (3)...Kerlone
Bevacizumab (1)...Avastin
Bexarotene (1)... Targretin
Bicalutamide (1)..Casodex
Bismuth (1).. Pepto-Bismol
Bisoprolol (1) .... Zebeta
Bleomycin (1) (3) (6) ....**Blenoxane**
Brinzolamide (1) ....Azopt
Bromocriptine (1) (3) (5) .... Parlodel
Bupropion (1)..Wellbutrin
Buspirone (1)..Buspar
Busulfan (1) (6) ....**Myleran**

C

Cabergoline (1) ....Dostinex
Capecitabine (1) .... Xeloda
Captopril (1) (3) .... Captopen
Carbamazepine (1) (5) .... Tegretol
Carbidopa (1) .... Sinemet
Carbimazole (3) (5)

Carboplatin (6) ....**Paraplatin**
Carmustine (1) (6) .... **Gliadel Wafer**
Carteolol (1) ....Cartrol
Carvedilol (1) ....Coreg
Celecoxib (1) ....Celebrex
Cerivastatin(1)
Cetirizine (1) ....Zyrtec
Cetuximab (1) .... Erbitux
Cevimeline (1)..Exovac
Chlorambucil (1) (6) .... **Leukeran**
Chloramphenicol (1) (5) .... Chloromycetin
Chlordiazepoxide (1)...Limbitrol
Chloroquine (1) (5) ....Aralen
Chlorothiazide (1) ....Aldochlor
Chlorotrianisene (1) .... Tace
Chlorpropamide (1)... Diabinese
Chlorthalidone (1)...Tenoretic
Chondroitin (1)...................... Chrondroitin Sulfate C
Cidofovir (1) (6) ....Forvade
Cimetidine (1) (3) (5) ....Tagamet
Cisplatin (1) (6) ....**Platinol**
Citalopram (1)...Celexa
Clofibrate (1) (3) ....Claripex
Clomiphene (1) .... Clomid
Clomipramine (1) .... Anafranil
Clonazepam (1)..Klonopin
Clonidine (1) .... Catapres
Colcemid (3)
Colchicine (1) (2) (3) (4) (5) (6)........................... **Colbenemid**
Corticosteroids (1)
Coumarin (3) (5)
Cyclobenzaprine (1)
Cyclophosphamide (1) (2) (3) (5) (6)........................**Cytoxan**
Cyclosporine (1)..Neoral
Cytarabine (1) (3) (6)......................................**Cytosar-U**

D

Dacarbazine (1) (3) (6)...............................**DTIC-Dome**
Dactinomycin (1) (3) (6)............................... Cosmegen
Dalteparin (1) (3) (6)......................................**Fragmin**
Danazol (1) (3) (6) .... Danocrine

Daunorubicin (1) (3) (6) ....**Cerubidine**
Delavirdine (1) .... Rescriptor
Desipramine (1) (3) .... Norpramin
Dexfenfluramine (1)
Dextran (3)
Diazoxide (1) .... Hyperstat
Dichloromethotrexate (3)
Diclofenac (1) .... Voltaren
Dicumarol (1) .... Dicumarol
Didanosine (1) .... Videx
Dideoxycytidine (1) .... Hivid
Diethylpropion (1) .... Tenuate
Diethylstilbestrol (1)
Diflunisal (1) .... Dolobid
Diltiazem (1) .... Teczem
Digoxin (1) .... Lanoxicaps
Disopyramide (1) .... Norpace
Dixyrazine (3)
Disopyramide (1)
Docetaxel (1) (6) ....**Taxotere**
Donepezil (1) .... Aricept
Dopamine (1) .... Dopastat
Doxazosin (1) .... Cardura
Doxepin (1) .... Sinequan; Zonalon (Topical)
Doxorubicin (1) (3) (5) (6) ....**Doxil**
Duloxetine (1) .... Cymbalta

E

Efavirenz (1) .... Sustiva
Elfornithine (1) .... Vania
Eletriptan (1) .... Relpax
Enalapril (1) (3) .... Vasotec
Endoxan (3)
Epinephrine (1) .... Adrenalin
Epirubicin (1) .... Ellence
Epoetin Alfa (1) .... Procrit
Escitalopram (1) .... Lexapro
Esmolol (1) .... Brevibloc
Estramustine (1) .... Emcyt
Estrogens (1)
Ethambutol (1) .... Myambutol
Ethionamide (1) .... Trecator SC

Ethosuximide (1) ....Zarontin
Etidronate (1)..Didronel
Etodolac (1).. Lodine
Etretinate (5)
Exemestane (1) ....Aromasin

F

Famotidine (1)..Pepcid
Felbamate (1) ....Felbatol
Fenofibrate (1) .... Tricor
Fenoprofen (1) .... Nalfon
Finasteride (1) .... Propecia
Flecainide (1) ....Tambocor
Floxuridine (3) ....FUDR
Fluconazole (1)... Diflucan
Fludarabine (1) (3).. Fludara
Fluorouracil (1) (3) (6)
Fluoxetine (1) (3)..Prozac
Fluoxymesterone (1)......................................Halostensin
Flurbiprofen (1) .... Ansaid
Fluvastatin (1) .... Lescol
Fluvoxamine (1) ....Luvox
Foscarnet (1) .... Foscavir

G

Gabapentin (1).. Neurontin
Ganciclovir(1) .... Cytovene
Gemcitabine (1) (6) ....**Gemzar**
Gemfibrozil (1).. Lopid
Glatiramer (1) .... Copaxone
Gold and gold compounds (1) (3)
Goserelin (1) ....Zoladex
Granisetron (1) ....Kytril
Granulocyte colony-stimulating factor (GCSF) (1) (6)
Guanethidine (1)..Ismelin
Guanfacine (1) .... Tenex

H

Haloperidol (1)..Haldol
Halothane (1) ....Fluothane
Heparin (1) (2) (3) (5) (6)................................... Hep-Flush
Hepatitis B Vaccine (3).......................... Recombivax HB
Hexamethylmelamine (5)

Hydantoin derivatives (1) ....Pilantin
Hydromorphone (1) .... Dilaudid
Hydroxycarbamide (6)
Hydroxychloroquine (1)..Plaquenil
Hydroxyurea (1) (3) (6) ....**Droxia**

I

Ibuprofen (1).. Advil
Idarubicin (1) (3) (6)..**Idamycin**
Ifosfamide (1) (3) (6)...**Ifex**
Immunoglobulin (3)
Imipramine (3)..Tofranil
Indinavir (1) (3) ....Crixivan
Indomethacin (1) (2) (4) ....Indocin
Interferons (1) (3) (6)   Interferons Beta (1)-A:Avonex
                                        Interferons Beta (1)-B:Betaseron
                                        Interferons Alfa (2): Infergen
Ipratropium (1) .... Combivent
Irinotecan (1) ....Camptosar
Isoniazid (1) ....Rifamate
Isotretinoin (1) (6).. Accutane
Itraconazole (1)... Sporanox

K

Ketoconazole (1)...Nizoral
Ketoprofen (1) .... Orudis

L

Labetalol (1) ....Normodyne
Lamivudine (1) .... Combivir
Lamotrigine (1)... Lamictal
Lansoprazole (1) ....Prevacid
Leflunomide (1) (6).. Arava
Letrozole (1)..Femara
Leucovorin (1)
Levodopa (3) (4) (5) .... Sinemet
Leuprolide (1) ....Lupron
Levamisole (1) .... Ergamisol
Levobetaxolol (1)... Betaxon
Levobunolol (1) (3) (6).. Betagan
Levodopa (1) (2) (3) .... L-dopa
Levothyroxine (1) .... Eltroxin
Liothyroxine (1).. Triostat

Lisinopril (1)..Zestril
Lithium (1)..Eskalith
Lithium carbonate (1) (2) (3) (6)
Lomustine (1) (3) (6) ....**CeeNU**
Loperamide (1) ....Maalox
Loratadine (1) ....Claritin
Lorazepam (1) ....Ativan
Losartan (1) ....Cozaar
Lovastatin (1) ....Advicor
Loxapine (1) ....Loxitane

M

Maprotiline (1)..Ludiomil
Mebendazole (1) (3)..................................Vermox
Mechloroethamine (1) (3) (6) ....**Mustargen**
Meclofenamate (1)
Medroxyprogesterone(1) (6)........**Depo-Provera**
Mefloquine (1) ....Lariam
Melphalan (1) (3) (6)................................**Alkeran**
Memantine (1) ....Namenda
Mepacrine (5)..Atabrine
Mephenytoin (1) ....Mesantoin
Mercaptopurine (1) (6) ....**Purinethol**
Mesalamine (1)..Asacol
Mesoridazine (1)..Serentil
Metformin (1) ....Glucovance
Methimazole (1) ....Tapazole
Methotrexate (1) (2) (3) (5) (6) ....Rheumatrex
Methsuximide (1) ....Celontin
Methyldopa (1) ....Aldoclor
Methylphenidate (1)......................................Ritalin
Methyltestosterone (1)............................Metandren
Methylthiouracil (3)
Methysergide (1) (3)................................Sansert
Metoprolol (1) (3) (5) ....Lopressor
Mexiletine (1)..Mexitil
Minocycline (1) (3)..................................Dynacin
Minoxidil (1) ....Rogaine
Misoprostol (1) (3) (6) ....**Cytotec**
Mitomycin (1) (6)................................**Mutamycin**
Mitotane (3)..Lysodren
Mitoxantrone (1) (6)................................Novantrone

Moexipril (1) .... Univasc
Mycophenolate (1)... CellCept

N

Nabumetone (1).. Relafen
Nadolol (1) (5) .... Corgard
Nalidixic acid (1) .... NegGram
Naltrexone (1)... Revex
Naproxen (1) .... Aleve
Naratriptan (1)... Amerge
Nefazodone (1) .... Serzone
Neomycin (1) .... Neosporin
Nifedipine (1)... Procardia
Nimodipine (1) .... Nimotop
Nisoldipine (1) .... Sular
Nitisinone (1).. Orfadin
Nitrofurantoin (1)... Furadantin
Nitrosureas (3)
Nortriptyline (1) .... Aventyl

O

Octreotide (1) .... Sandostatin
Olanzapine (1)... Zyprexa
Omeprazole (1).. Prilosec
Ondansetron (1) .... Zofran
Oral Contraceptives (1) (3) (4)
Oxaliplatin (1)... Eloxatin
Oxcarbazepine (1) .... Trileptal

P

Paclitaxel (6) ....**Taxol**
Pantoprazole (1)... Protonix
Paramethadione (1) .... Paradione
Paroxetine (1)... Paxil
Peg-interferon Alfa-(2)B (1)
PEG-Intron (1)
Pegfilgrastim (1).. Neulasta
Penbutolol (1) .... Levatol
Penicillamine (1) (5)... Cuprimine
Penicillins (1)
Pentosan (1) .... Elmiron
Pentostatin (1) (6)...**Nipent**
Pergolide (1).. Permax

Phensuximide (1) .... Milontin
Phentermine (1) .... Fastin
Phenytoin (1) .... Dilantin
Pindolol (1) .... Visken
Pirbuterol (1) .... Maxair
Piroxicam (1) .... Feldene
Pravastatin (1) .... Pravachol
Prazepam (1) .... Centrax
Prazosin (1) .... Minizide
Probenecid (1) .... Benemid
Procarbazine (1) (3) (6) .... **Procan**
Progestins (1)
Proguanil (3)
Propafenone (1) .... Rythmol
Propranolol (1) (2) (3) (4) (5) .... Inderal
Propylthiouracil (1) (3) .... Propylthiouracil
Protriptyline (1) .... Vivactil
Pyridostigmine bromide (3) (5)
Pyrimethamine (1) .... Daraprim

Q

Quazepam (1) .... Doral
Quinacrine (1) (2) (4) .... Atabrine
Quinidine (1) .... Cardioquin
Quinine (2) .... Legatrin

R

Rabeprazole (1) (6) .... Aciphex
Ramipril (1) .... Altace
Ranitidine (1) .... Zantac
Retinol, Retinoids (3) (4) (5)
Ribavirin (1) .... Rebetol
Riluzole (1)
Risperidone (1) .... Risperdal
Ritonavir (1) .... Norvir
Rivastigmine (1) .... Exelon
Ropinirole (1) .... Requip

S

Saquinavir (1) .... Fortovase
Selegiline (1) .... Eldepryl
Selenium (1) .... Head & Shoulders
Sertraline (1) .... Zoloft

Simvastatin (1) ....Zocor
Sodium cromoglycate (1) .... Crolom
Sotalol (1) ....Betapace
Sparfloxacin (1) ....Zagam
Spironolactone (1) ....Aldactone
St. John's Wort (1)
Stanozolol (1) .... Winstrol
Sulfasalazine (1) (3) (5) .... Azulfidine
Sulfisoxazole (1) ....Pediazole
Sulindac (1)... Clinoril

T

Tacrine (1) .... Cognex
Tacrolimus (1) .... Protopic
Tamoxifen (1) ....Nolvadex
Terbinafine (1) (6) ....Lamisil
Testosterone (1) (2)... Androderm
Thalidomide (1) .... Contergan
Thallium (2) (4)
Thioguanine (1) (6)................................... **Contegram**
Thioridazine (1) .... Mellaril
Thiotepa (1) (6)..**Thioplex**
Thiothixene (1) .... Navane
Thiouracil (2) (3)
Tiagabine (1) ....Gabitril
Timolol (1) (3) (6) ....Betimol
Tinazaparin (1)..Innohep
Tiopronin (1)... Thiola
Tocainide (1) .... Tonocard
Tolcapone (1) ....Tasmar
Topiramate (1) ....Topamax
Topotecan (1) (6) .... Hycamtin
Trazodone (1) ....Desyrel
Tranylcypromine (3) .... Parnate
Triazolam (1) ....**Halcion**
Triethylenethiophosphoramide (3)
Trimethadione (1) (2) (5) .... Tridione
Trimipramine (1)...Surmontil
Triparanol (3)
Triptorelin (1).. Trelstar

U

Urofollitropin (1) ....Bravelle
Ursodiol (1) .... Actigall

V

Valdecoxib (1) .... Bextra
Valproic acid (1) (3) (6) ....Depacon
Valproate sodium (2) (5)
Vasopressin (1) (6) ....**Pitressin**
Venlafaxine (1) ....Effexor
Varapamil (1).. Covera-HS
Vinblastine (1) (3) (6) .... **Velban**
Vincristine (1) (3) (6) ....**Oncovin**
Vinorelbine (1) (6)`Navelbine
Vitamin A (1) (3) (4).. Aquasol A
Voriconazole (1)..Vfend

W

Warfarin (6) .... Coumadin

Z

Zalcitabine (1)...Hivid
Zaleplon (1) ....Sonata
Zidovudine (1) .... Combivir
Ziprasidone (1)... Geodon
Zonisamide (1) ....Zonegran

GLOSSARY

A

Aldactone: Brand name for spironolactone, a prescription high blood pressure medication that may also be prescribed to treat hair loss in women.

Alopecia: Medical term for hair loss.

Alopecia areata: An auto immune disease in which the body's immune system attacks certain hair follicles, resulting in patchy hair loss, usually on the scalp. The bald patches may regrow hair within a few months, or the hair loss may persist for many years.

Alopecia totalis: A variation of alopecia areata in which all scalp hair is lost.

Alopecia reduction: Commonly called a scalp reduction. A surgical procedure in which a portion of the bald scalp is removed and the edges are pulled together and sutured closed.

Alopecia universalis: A variation of alopecia areata in which all body hair is lost.

Anagen phase: Growth phase of a hair follicle, during which the hair shaft grows about a half inch per month. The anagen phase of scalp hair follicles typically lasts four to six years. Hair follicles in other areas such as the eyelashes, have shorter anagen phases, resulting in shorter hairs.

Androgens: A class of hormones commonly called "male" hormones, because of their higher concentration in adult men, than adult women. Testosterone and Dihydrotestosterone (DHT) are both androgens.

Androgenetic alopecia: The medical term for inherited hair loss. Androgenetic refers to an inherited sensitivity to certain androgens, specifically DHT, which signals susceptible hair follicles to stop growing. Alopecia is the medical term for hair loss.

Appliance: A common industry name for a hairpiece.

Autograft: A surgical transfer of tissue from one part of an organism to another part of the same organism. Hair transplants are autograft procedures, as the patient is always his or her own "donor".

Autoimmune disease: A medical disorder in which an organism's immune system turns against itself. The cause of most autoimmune disorders is unknown, and there may be periods when the white blood cells attack certain tissue, and other periods where there are no symptoms. Alopecia areata is an autoimmune disease in which the rapidly dividing cells in the hair follicle bulb are attacked. Treatments include steroid hormones and other non-steroid anti-inflammatory medications.

B

Bulb: The part of the hair follicle that lies deepest in the skin, surrounding the hair matrix and dermal papilla cells, which rapidly divide to produce the hair shaft.

Bulge: An area located near the middle of the hair follicle, below the sebaceous (oil) gland and near the attachment point for the arrector pili muscle (the tiny muscle that allows hairs to "stand on end"). The bulge is believed to be where hair follicle stem cells are located, which begin the process of rebuilding the hair follicle as each new growth phase starts.

C

Castration: The removal of sex organs in men or women, either by surgical or chemical means. Removal of testicles in men decreases testosterone levels to such a degree that the enzyme 5-alpha-reductase is only able to convert a small amount of testosterone into DHT, and as a result of the low levels of DHT, the DHT-sensitive hair follicles don't get the message to stop growing new hairs. In 420 BC Hippocrates, the Father of Modern Medicine, observed that castration before puberty prevented baldness. Castration after puberty will stop further hair loss, but will not help regrow hair that was lost earlier. The side effects of this hair loss treatment method are severe.

Catagen phase: The regression phase of the cycle of hair growth. It follows the anagen (growth) phase, and precedes the telogen (resting) phase. During the catagen phase, the hair stops growing and the lower portion of the hair follicle begins to disintegrate.

Chemotherapy: A type of treatment commonly used after cancer surgery or radiation treatment that uses powerful chemicals to interfere with tumor growth. The chemicals also affect some healthy tissue, especially fast growing cells such as those in hair follicles, resulting in temporary hair loss.

Cortisone: A steroid hormone often used to treat alopecia areata. It is believed to confuse the white blood cells mistakenly attacking the hair follicles, and thereby allow the hair follicles to recover and grow hair again.

D

Dandruff: Dandruff is a scalp condition characterized by excessive scaling and skin flake shedding. Dandruff is sometimes accompanied by itching, and often oiliness, but without visible redness or inflammation. Although the exact cause of dandruff is not completely understood, the condition is associated with an increase in the population of certain microorganisms that naturally occur on the scalp, including Pityrosporum ovale, a yeast-like fungus that lives in the oil glands and hair follicles on the scalp. The cause of the increase in the population of Pityrosporum ovale is not well understood, and dandruff conditions often change over time, even without treatment. Dandruff does not cause hair loss.

Dermal papilla: A variety of rapidly dividing cells inside the hair bulb. The dermal papilla cells connect with the bundle of blood capillaries that nourish the hair follicle.

Dermatologist: A medical doctor who is trained to treat conditions affecting the skin, hair and nails.

DHT: Abbreviation for Dihydrotestosterone.

Dihydrotestosterone: A naturally occurring hormone in the blood that in men and women with an inherited tendency for hair loss, signals hair follicles sensitive to dihydrotestosterone to stop growing new hairs. The enzyme 5-alpha-reductase converts some testosterone in the blood into dihydrotestosterone.

Donor area: The area on the scalp selected for having hair follicles that are DHT-resistant, and will likely continue growing new hairs for the individual's lifetime. The donor area is typically the back of the scalp, and the sides extending behind the ears. The donor area is the part of the scalp that in "pattern baldness" does not get bald.

Dutasteride: A 5-alpha-reductase inhibitor medication that inhibits both type-I and type-II 5-alpha-reductase.

E

Enzyme: A type of protein that alters other proteins, and organic molecules. The enzyme 5-alpha-reductase converts the hormone protein testosterone into dihydrotestosterone (DHT).

Estrogen: A class of hormones commonly called "female" hormones, because of their higher concentration in adult women, than adult men. Estrogens are the active ingredient in birth control pills, and are also used treat symptoms of menopause. High estrogen levels in the blood of women can interfere with their DHT-sensitive hair follicles from getting the message to stop growing new hairs. When estrogen levels decline, the message begins to get through, and thinning hair can result.

Extension: A type of partial wig that adds long hairs to shorter existing hair.

F

Female pattern hair loss: The counterpart to the more common phrase "male pattern baldness," female pattern hair loss describes the typical pattern of hair loss suffered by women who have DHT-sensitive hair follicles. Typically women do not get clear bald patches or receding hairlines, but their hair does get thin on top and to a lesser degree on the sides and back of the scalp. The donor area for women electing to have hair transplants is the same as for men: the back of the scalp.

Ferritin: An iron-binding protein necessary for red blood cell function. A low ferritin level in the blood is an indication of iron-deficiency anemia.

Finasteride: The generic name for the active ingredient in Propecia. 5-alpha-reductase: an enzyme that converts testosterone in the blood into dihydrotestosterone (DHT). There are two types of 5-alpha-reductase, called type-I and type-II. Medications that interfere with 5-alpha-reductase can stop hair loss.

Follicle: The miniature organ in the skin that grows hair. Each follicle grows a single hair during a growth phase, and then the follicle regresses and shrinks in size, sheds the hair, rests for a period of time, and then grows back to full size as it begins a new growth phase.

Follicular unit: A micrograft hair transplant term that refers to naturally occurring clusters of hair follicles. Follicular unit micrografts contain intact clusters of hair follicles which produce natural-looking clusters of hair when they are transplanted. A follicular unit may be a single follicle, or may have two, three, or more follicles.

Full size graft: A circular skin graft about the size of a split pea, containing seven to fifteen hair follicles. Full size grafts were the standard size graft for hair transplants before micrografting techniques improved the survival rate of smaller grafts. Full size grafts are sometimes called "plugs" by those not in the hair restoration surgery business.

G

General anesthesia: Medication that puts the patient "to sleep" during a surgical procedure. General anesthesia has greater risk of medical complications than local anesthesia, and may require a doctor specially trained in anesthesiology to administer the medication.

Gene: A portion of a DNA molecule that contains instructions for making a particular protein, such as a hormone.

Genetic: Inherited, as a result of receiving the same genes as one's ancestors.

H

Hair addition: A partial wig constructed of human or synthetic hair typically used to add the appearance of length to existing hair. Hair additions are often attached by a comb or by weaving into existing hair.

Hairpiece: A partial wig constructed of human or synthetic hair attached to a lightweight mesh base. Hairpieces are constructed so that their hairs blend in with the remaining growing hairs on the user. Hairpieces may be attached by a variety of methods, however double-sided tape and liquid adhesives are most commonly used.

Hair: A long cylinder of dead cells containing high concentrations of keratin protein.

Hair Replacement: A common industry name for a hairpiece.

Hair shaft: A hair.

Hair transplant: A surgical procedure in which tissue containing hair follicles from a donor site such as the back of the scalp are selected for resistance to genetic hair loss and are surgically removed, cut into grafts containing one or more follicles, and the grafts are then placed into recipient sites in the locations such as the hairline and top of the scalp. The transplanted hair follicles establish new connections to the blood supply, and begin growing new hairs, just as they would have at their original location. By redistributing the patient's hair follicles, hair transplants very effectively achieve the illusion of a fuller head of hair.

Hirsutism: Excessive body hair in a male pattern. Hirsutism can affect both men and women, and may be caused by heredity, hormone imbalances, or medications.

Hormone: A type of protein that travels through the bloodstream to signal specific cellular activity.

Hypertrichosis: A medical term for excessive hair growth.

I

Implants: In contrast to transplants of live hair follicle grafts, implants refer to surgical placement of synthetic fibers, or strands of hair, into the scalp. The procedure results in severe immune response as the body attacks the foreign substance, and implants have been banned in the United States. They are still legal to perform in some other countries, however.

J - K

Keratin: A structural protein found in hair, and also skin, nails, and tooth enamel.

L

Local anesthetic: Medication injected at a specific location to numb the sensation of pain. In surgical procedures involving local anesthetic, the patient is awake.

M

Male pattern baldness: A common way of describing the appearance of androgenetic alopecia, the tendency for inherited hair loss in men. The pattern typically begins with a receding hairline or thinning at the crown, or both. Eventually the hairline recedes, and the top of the head becomes bald, leaving only a fringe of hair at the back of the scalp and behind the ears. The hair follicles in the bald areas are genetically programmed at birth to be sensitive to DHT in the blood, and slowly stop producing new hairs. The hair follicles in the scalp on the back and sides are genetically programmed to be DHT-resistant.

Menopause: The end of menstruation and reproductive capability in women as a result of decreased estrogen production. Typically women begin perimenopause around age forty, and by age fifty-five to fifty-eight most women are in menopause. Decreased estrogen levels can allow DHT-sensitive hair follicles to stop growing new hairs, and result in thin hair in post-menopausal women.

Micrograft: A skin graft about the size of half a grain of rice, typically containing one to three hair follicles. Micrografts are the standard graft for hair transplants today. Micrografts that are comprised of naturally occurring clusters of hair follicles are called follicular unit micrografts.

Minoxidil: The generic name for the active ingredient in Rogaine lotion.

Mitosis: The process of cell division for growth and repair of tissue.

N - O

Oral contraceptive: Birth control pills. Oral contraceptives contain estrogens, which can help some women with declining estrogen levels and a genetic tendency for hair loss to keep their hair.

P

Plugs: A common name for full size hair transplant grafts.

Prostate gland: A small organ in men only that surrounds the neck of the bladder, and that secretes various enzymes including type-II 5-alpha-reductase.

Propecia: Currently the most effective hair loss treatment medication. Propecia tablets contain the medication finasteride.

Q - R

Recipient area: The portion of the scalp where hair transplant grafts are placed. The recipient area includes bald and thin areas, as well as areas that are likely to become thin as a result of future hair loss.

Rogaine: Brand name for the lotion form of the hair loss treatment medication minoxidil.

S

Scalp reduction: Sometimes called an alopecia reduction, it refers to the removal of the bald scalp. A surgical procedure in which a portion of the bald scalp is removed and the edges are pulled together and sutured closed.

Spironolactone: The generic name for the active ingredient in the medication Aldactone. Spironolactone is a potent anti-androgen, and binds to DHT receptor sites on hair follicles, thereby blocking DHT from getting its hair loss message to the follicles.

Stem cells: Undifferentiated cells that produce intermediate cells called transient amplifying cells, which in turn produce specialized cells as the organism needs them.

T

Telogen: The resting stage of the cycle of hair growth.

Testosterone: The most well known androgen hormone, found in both men and women, but in higher concentrations in men. Some testosterone in the blood is converted by 5-alpha-reductase into dihydrotestosterone (DHT), which signals DHT-sensitive hair follicles to stop growing new hairs.

Topical: A medication applied to the surface of the skin, in liquid, cream, ointment, gel, foam, paste, tincture or lotion form.

Toupee: An old-fashioned name for a hairpiece.

Traction alopecia: A type of hair loss that results from pulling on the hair, typically from tight hairstyles such as cornrows and ponytails. The hair loss is temporary; repeated pulling will prematurely age the follicles and could eventually result in permanent hair loss.

Trichotillomania: A psychological disorder in which a person pulls out his or her own hair. The condition is typically seen in young children who pull on their hair at night during sleep, but can also occur in adults and while awake. The hair loss is temporary. Repeated pulling will prematurely age the follicles and could eventually result in permanent hair loss.

U

Unit: A common industry name for a hairpiece.

V - W

Weave: A type of hairpiece that is attached to the scalp by weaving the growing hairs through the edge of the hairpiece. Weaves do not involve the use of adhesives, but must be reattached after a few weeks as the attachment hairs grow out or become loose.

Wig: An artificial hair device that completely covers the scalp, and temporarily replaces whatever hair the user has (if any) with synthetic or human hair that makes up the wig. Wigs may be attached by a variety of methods, including adhesives, double-sided tape, and for users with no hair on their scalp, by vacuum fit.

Bibliography

Clinical Dermatology
    2nd Edition, Habif, Thomas P.
    CV Mosby Company
    St. Louis 1990

Hair Transplantation
    4th Edition, Unger, Walter, Shapiro, Ron
    Marcell Dekker, 2004

Dermatology Moschella and Hurley
    Moschella, Samuel L., Hurley, Harry J. (eds)
    WB Saunders Company
    Philadelphia 1985

Diseases of the Hair and Scalp
    Rook A., Dawber RPR (eds)
    Blackwell Scientific Publications
    Oxford 1991

Disorders of Hair Growth
    Olsen, Elise A. (ed)
    McGraw Hill Inc
    New York 1994

Drug Eruption Reference Manual 2005
    Litt, Jerome Z.
    Eleventh Edition
    Taylor and Francis 2005

Propecia The Hair-Growth Breakthrough
    Seiden, Othniel J.
    Prima Publishing
    Rocklin, CA 1998

The Intelligent Man's Guide to Hair Transplants
    Unger, Walter
    Contemporary Books
    Chicago 1979

What You Can Do about Chronic Hair Loss
    Bruning, Nancy
    Dell Publishing 1993

INDEX